The Directory

Essential Oils

South Tr

THE DIRECTORY
OF ESSENTIAL OILS

Wanda Sellar

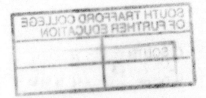

SAFFRON WALDEN
THE C.W. DANIEL COMPANY LIMITED

First published in Great Britain in 1992
by The C.W. Daniel Company Limited,
1 Church Path, Saffron Walden,
Essex CB10 1JP, England

Revised Edition 1992
Reprinted 1993
Revised Edition 1994

© Wanda Sellar 1992

ISBN 0 85207 239 2

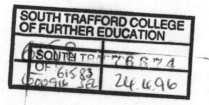
Designed by Dale Dawson
Production in association with
Book Production Consultants plc, Cambridge
Typeset by Cambridge Photosetting Services
Printed and bound by St Edmundsbury Press, Bury St Edmunds, Suffolk.

Dedication

For Pamela

Contents

Acknowledgements

My thanks to the Enfield Library and to friends and colleagues who have aided and abetted my labours, in particular Dr Vivian Lunny, Jean Goodall, Lindsay Bamfield and Christina Bennett. I am grateful too to the following essential oil companies who lent a helpful hand; Fleur Aromatherapy, Ronald Hagman Laboratories, Phoenix Products and Butterbur & Sage Ltd.

The Publisher wishes to thank and acknowledge the following companies for the loan of the bottles appearing on the front cover: Atlantic Aromatics, Bodytreats Limited, Butterbur and Sage London, Culpeper Limited, Fleur Aromatherapy, Fragrant Earth Company, Ronald Hagman Limited, Neals Yard Remedies and Tisserand Aromatherapy Products Limited. Especial thanks to Phoenix Products of Southall, Middlesex for their generous loan of glassware and oils.

Introduction

The healing art of Aromatherapy needs little introduction nowadays. So I will be brief. Other books set out application methods of essential oils. This one just describes their character and the various ways they can help to enhance the Mind and Body and in so doing perhaps they can lift the Spirit too.

Each essential oil is categorised under different headings so the relevant information is immediately to hand. A compilation such as this one, can serve as an aid to the Aromatherapist when choosing appropriate oils for treatment. Yet since each person is a wondrous mixture of individual qualities, the therapeutic claims associated with each oil can often be more of a promise than a cure. Perhaps finally, healing comes through the therapist's own intuition in pairing the oil with the client.

Ailments listed which are of a severe nature should of course only be treated in collaboration with a qualified medical doctor.

Though massage is the usual method of treatment in Aromatherapy – between 1 and 3 drops of essential oil to a teaspoon of base oil – some entries here may not be appropriate to this healing medium. The section headed Precautions usually indicates this, but it's important to remember that Aromatherapy is a very subtle form of healing and just a little goes a very long way. Some essential oils are listed more through general interest and perhaps are too potent to include within the Aromatherapists' pharmacopoeia. This is mentioned too.

The 'Notes' whether High, Middle or Base have not always found universal agreement, neither have the planetary rulerships. But maybe what we have here is a good starting point rather than the last word. In the same way the section under Blends is just a helpful guide in selecting combinations though personal preference can be paramount in healing. There is also a separate section on Blends at the back of the book, indicating possible combinations. Each group is said to blend well together as well as those adjacent to it. The chemical constituents also just hint at the complexity of each essential oil.

It was the History category which really brought the oils to life for me, though naturally many of the tales belonged more to the plant rather than the essential oil. Ginger and Black Pepper were very assertive though others like Chamomile and Violet showed a gentler face.

A Glossary at the back provides a handy cross-reference for the Properties. Most of the main oils are included.

London 1992

AMYRIS

Plant/Part	:	Tree/Wood
Latin Name	:	Amyris balsamifera
Family	:	Rutaceae
Note	:	Base
Planet	:	?
Extraction	:	Distillation

AROMA: Dry, burnt wood fragrance.

FEATURES: Amyris grows wild on the mountain slopes of Haiti. Often found in small thickets, it is an evergreen with lovely white flowers though it is the bark which emits the valuable resinous fluid. Acclaimed as the West Indian Sandalwood yet it does not belong to the same family i.e. Santalaceae. Different regions of production seem to produce a slightly different type of oil, the quality of which largely depends upon moisture content and age of tree. If the wood is ground too finely, there is a reduction of oil.

HISTORY & MYTH: The wood burns like a candle due to its plentiful oil content hence its other popular pseudonym Candlewood. Not surprisingly it was also chopped up for firewood. It was a familiar sight along the sea-shores of Haiti at night since fishermen used the twigs as a torch to catch sea crabs. Similarly villagers travelling at night-time would light their way with Amyris twigs when they brought farm produce from their mountain dwellings to the cities. Its durable quality found a practical use as fence posts too.

Prior to the Second World War, large quantities of small logs were exported from Venezuela, Haiti and Jamaica for distillation chiefly in Germany. The Properties are said to be similar to that of East Indian Sandalwood which oil it has been known to adulterate. Principal use has been as a fixative in perfumes and as an ingredient of soaps and cosmetics.

CONSTITUENTS: Cadinene, Cadinole, Caryophyllene (Sesquiterpenes).

PROPERTIES: Antiseptic, Antiphlogistic, Antispasmodic, Aphrodisiac, Expectorant, Hypotensive, Sedative.

PRECAUTIONS: A lingering aroma which might not please all. Otherwise other contraindications unknown.

MIND: Possibly effective in easing nervous tension.

BODY: We start with an oil about which little is known except its colourful and interesting history. Therapeutics are little more than guess-work based on its similarity to Sandalwood and Sesquiterpene content.

This indicates a soothing, sedative quality which is also associated with Base notes – Amyris being used as a fixative in perfumes. Its antispasmodic nature ties in with its calming character and like Sandalwood, could well ease coughs and chest complaints. Possibly hypotensive too, helping to bring down blood pressure.

Since most oils are antiseptic, no doubt Amyris also has this quality and may help to ward off infection. The strength of its potency in this regard is however, uncertain.

Is it possible that like Sandalwood, it could well have an effect on urinary complaints? However, its competence as an aphrodisiac must, no doubt, be left to personal investigation!

EFFECT ON SKIN: Antiphlogistic qualities are often characteristic of Sesquiterpenes so its possible that Amyris may well have a soothing effect on inflammatory conditions. However, with its 'burnt wood' aroma could this in fact also point to a 'drying' effect on oily skin conditions?

BLENDS: Benzoin, Clary Sage, Elemi, Frankincense, Galbanum, Geranium, Jasmine, Lavender, Melissa, Rose, Rosewood, Ylang Ylang.

ANGELICA

Plant/Part	:	Herb/seeds/roots
Latin Name	:	Angelica archangelica
Family	:	Umbelliferae
Note	:	Base
Planet	:	Sun
Extraction	:	Distillation

AROMA: Sweet, herbaceous and a little musky.

FEATURES: A water loving herb often found nearby rivers and streams. Grows quite tall with large, broad pointed leaves dividing into smaller leaflets adorned by tiny greenish-white flowers. Many varieties of Angelica grow over Northern Europe as well as Iceland, Greenland and central Russia and the oil is often obtained from England and Belgium.

HISTORY & MYTH: Some time during the 16th century, Angelica came out of North Africa and into the warmer climes of Europe. Since first flowering on 8th May – St Michael the Archangel's Day – it has been used in mystical rituals. Perhaps not surprisingly, it was frequently grown in monasteries and known in those ancient dwellings as 'Angel Grass'.

Popular French liqueurs such as Chartreuse and Benedictine include this delightful herb. It grew to be a favourite garden plant, and was widely regarded as an antidote to the Plague. 'Angelica Water' formed part of a royal prescription and was published in pamphlet form by the College of Physicians in 1665, the year of London's Great Plague. The old medic Paracelsus esteemed it highly and reckoned it to be a cure-all. Often used to flavour gin and perfumes and traditionally candied for cake decoration and confectionary.

CHEMICAL CONSTITUENTS: Borneol, Linalool (Alcohols), Bergaptene (Lactone), Limonene, Phellandrene, Pinene (Terpenes).

PROPERTIES: Antispasmodic, Aphrodisiac, Carminative, Diuretic, Emmenagogue, Expectorant, Hepatic, Stomachic, Stimulant, Sudorific, Tonic.

PRECAUTIONS: Excessive use may over stimulate the nervous system possibly causing insomnia. Could be phototoxic, i.e. causing irritation when the skin is exposed to the sun. Best avoided in pregnancy and some say diabetes.

MIND: A fillip to the nervous system quickly relieving exhaustion and stress. Promotes a feeling of balance and appears to revitalise a tired mind and a flagging heart. Gives incentive to face difficult problems.

BODY: Its tonic action has a potent healing effect on the body particularly at the start of treatment by strengthening the constitution. It invigorates the lymphatic system, speeds up cleansing through its sweating action, drains fluids and relieves the body of poisons especially after a long illness.

Helps with indigestion, flatulence, dyspepsia (feeling of nausea and discomfort), stomach ulcers and colic. Stimulates appetite and may help with anorexia nervosa. Said to be a tonic to the liver and spleen. A urinary antiseptic hence useful in cystitis.

Its expectorant qualities work on feverish colds, chronic bronchitis and pleurisy. Seems to ease nervous asthma, shortness of breath and smokers cough as well as restoring sense of smell. Appears to be a general tonic to the lungs.

Said to encourage production of oestrogen thereby regulating menstruation and easing painful periods as well as helping to expel afterbirth. Reputedly useful with male and female infertility.

Controls uric acid and may be beneficial to rheumatic conditions and arthritis as well as gout and sciatica.

A speedy pain reliever – headaches, migraines and toothache may all benefit by its action.

And last but not least, neutralises snake bites!

EFFECT ON SKIN: A good skin tonic and also said to be anti-inflammatory which might be beneficial to various skin problems. Reputedly deals with fungal growths.

BLENDS: Basil, Chamomile, Geranium, Grapefruit, Lavender, Lemon, Mandarin.

ANISEED

Plant/Part	:	Herb/Seeds
Latin Name	:	Pimpinella anisum
Family	:	Umbelliferae
Note	:	Top to Middle
Planet	:	Sun?
Extraction	:	Distillation

AROMA: Pungent, liquorice-like, very warming.

FEATURES: The Middle East first gave us Aniseed and its now found in the warmer parts of Europe as well as North Africa and the USA. Cultivated to about two feet it has delicate feathery leaves with tiny white blossoms. The greyish-brown seeds are crushed before distillation increasing the oil yield. Low temperatures tend to solidify the oil and it may need to be hand-warmed before use.

HISTORY & MYTH: Revered by ancient civilisations, particularly in the Middle East. The practical Egyptians used Aniseed in bread-making probably for its carminative properties. The Romans hailed it as an aphrodisiac! They also used the seeds for a spicy cake known as 'mustaceus'. The Greeks recognised its calmative influence on the digestive tract. More recently it has been used in liqueurs and cordials such as pernod and absinthe. In India the seeds are chewed to sweeten the breath. Has been used an as ingredient in toothpastes and mouthwashes.

CHEMICAL CONSTITUENTS: Anisic (Aldehyde), Anethole, Methylchavicol (Phenols), Limonene (Terpene).

PROPERTIES: Antiemetic, Antispasmodic, Aphrodisiac, Cardiac, Carminative, Digestive, Diuretic, Expectorant, Galactagogue, Insecticide, Laxative, Parasiticide, Parturient, Pectoral, Stimulant, Stomachic.

PRECAUTIONS: A very potent oil, not often used in massage as skin sensitisation may occur. Generally a stimulant but excessive use could cause sluggishness. In extreme cases possibility of circulatory problems and cerebral congestion. Certainly should be avoided in pregnancy and perhaps altogether.

MIND: Could invigorate a tired mind.

BODY: Well known for its effect on the digestive system. May be helpful with dyspepsia, colic and flatulence. Seems to quell vomiting and nausea especially of nervous origin. Gets things moving by stimulating peristalsis. Apparently helpful with oliguria (low quantity of urine).

Has been used as a stimulant in cardiac fatigue though at the same time could ease palpitations. A general tonic to the circulatory system and respiratory tract. Used in lung and heart disease generally and may have a good effect on asthma and breathing difficulties. Appears to help with colds due to its warming properties.

Sexual problems such as impotence and frigidity may be helped – the Romans thought so anyway! Stimulates the glands and its oestrogen content seems to have a regulating effect on the reproductive system. Also calms menstrual pain, aids quick delivery in childbirth and stimulates the flow of milk in nursing mothers.

Migraine and vertigo sufferers benefit and those prone to hangovers!

EFFECT ON SKIN: Said to control lice and the 'itch mite' a cause of scabies. Generally has a reputation for dealing with infectious skin diseases.

BLENDS: Amyris, Bay, Cardamom, Caraway, Cedarwood, Coriander, Dill, Fennel, Galbanum, Mandarin, Petitgrain, Rosewood.

ANISE-STAR

Plant/Part	:	Tree/Fruit
Latin Name	:	Illicium verum
Family	:	Magnoliaceae
Note	:	Top
Planet	:	Sun?
Extraction	:	Distillation

AROMA: Penetrating, pungent, similar to Aniseed.

FEATURES: This ancient and exotic evergreen tree comes from East Asia and reaches to about thirty feet. Preferring its native land it eschews other locations. Yellow flowers and star-shaped fruits adorn a white bark. The fruits are distilled in their fresh green state, the oil having a similar though stronger aroma to Aniseed. Anise-Star is derived from Chinese Anise and sometimes referred to as 'Anise Vert' due to its green colouring. There is a Japanese variety (Illicium religiosum) which is poisonous.

HISTORY & MYTH: The village industries of Indo-China included essential oil of Anise-Star. Though it is often said to be of inferior quality to Aniseed the Chinese were still quite keen to use it as an ingredient of their medicines. Certainly it was a popular aperitif and was sometimes ground in tea and coffee to sweeten the breath. Meat dishes such as pork and duck were flavoured with Anise-Star and it found a way into sweet dishes as well. English navigators brought it to Europe in 16th century and was soon much in demand for flavouring liqueurs in France, Germany and Italy.

CHEMICAL CONSTITUENTS: Cineole (Ketone), Anethole, Safrole (Phenol), Carene, Cymene, Dipentene, Limonene, Pinene, Phellandrene (Terpenes).

PROPERTIES: Carminative, Diuretic, Expectorant, Stimulant, Stomachic.

PRECAUTIONS: A potent oil and may over-stimulate the nervous system – best avoided by people prone to allergies. Does not generally have a widespread use in Aromatherapy, and it may be best to avoid it all together.

MIND: Generally stimulating effects.

BODY: Seems to do an all-purpose job on the digestive system due to its strongly carminative nature. Settles the stomach and dispels flatulence and relieves feelings of nausea. Effective against constipation by stimulating peristalsis. Its beneficial action on the gut generally is probably the basis for its soothing effect on hernias.

Its diuretic properties could help with bladder problems typically cystitis and oliguria.

A warming effect on colds points to a beneficial action on the respiratory system. Has a reputation for soothing sore throats and chest infections. Apparently helpful with lumbago, a rheumatic condition usually resulting from cold weather.

Also said to encourage production of oestrogen and could be useful with pre menstrual tension, painful periods and acts as a regulator of menstruation.

EFFECT ON SKIN: ?

BLENDS: Caraway, Cardamom, Coriander, Cypress, Dill, Fennel, Ginger, Mandarin, Petitgrain, Rosewood.

BASIL

Plant/Part	:	Herb/Flowering tops and leaves
Latin Name	:	Ocimum Basilicum
Family	:	Labiatae
Note	:	Top
Planet	:	Mars
Extraction	:	Distillation

AROMA: Very clear, sweet and slightly spicy.

FEATURES: The many varieties of Basil originate from Asia and the Pacific islands. The broadly oval and pointed green leaves support lovely purple-white flowers on a sixteen inch stem. Swarms of bees hover around this plant in summer. North Africa, France, Cyprus and the Seychelles give us the essential oil though European Basil is said to be the best quality.

HISTORY & MYTH: Basilicum is from the Greek word 'Basilicos' meaning 'royal'. A mix-up with the Latin 'Basilicus' referring to serpent briefly gave Basil an unsavory reputation. Unscrupulous Magicians thought they could create scorpions by crushing Basil between two stones. Wiser Indian folklore held Basil sacred to Krishna and Vishnu, endowing it with protective qualities. Indeed some Indian tribes chew Basil leaves before taking part in religious ceremonies to gain inspiration. It is used extensively in ayurvedic medicine.

The Chinese favoured it for many centuries as a useful medicine and it seems to have a reputation for curing epilepsy. It soared in popularity during 2nd World War when spices were hard to come by. The essential oil is used in perfumery.

CHEMICAL CONSTITUENTS: Linalool (Alcohol), Borneone, Camphor, Cineole (Ketones), Methylchavicol, Eugenol (Phenols), Ocimene, Pinene, Sylvestrene (Terpenes).

PROPERTIES: Analgesic, Antidepressant, Antiseptic, Antispasmodic, Antivenomous, Aphrodisiac, Bacteriacide, Carminative, Cephalic, Digestive, Emmenagogue, Expectorant, Febrifuge, Galactogue, Insecticide, Nervine, Stomachic, Sudorific, Tonic, Restorative, Stimulant, Vermifuge.

PRECAUTIONS: Usually stimulating but has a stupefying effect when used in excess. An emmenagogue so perhaps best to avoid in pregnancy. Also might be irritant to people with sensitive skin.

MIND: A good tonic for the nerves, especially when feeling fragile, sharpening the senses and encouraging concentration. Apparently calms hysteria and nervous disorders yet seems to have an uplifting effect on depression.

BODY: First rate with headaches and migraine, probably due to its cephalic properties. Said to revive fainting spells and temporary paralysis. It is claimed to get rid of nasal polyps and earache. Could reduce allergies since it has an effect on the adrenal cortex which controls allergies related to stress.

Basil seems to have a beneficial action on the respiratory tract and is often used for sinus congestion, asthma, bronchitis, emphysema (excess air in tissues), influenza and whooping cough. Restores sense of smell lost through catarrh.

Also effective in digestive disorders such as vomiting, gastric spasm, nausea, dyspepsia (discomfort in upper digestive tract), and hiccups. Seems to cleanse the intestines and kidneys through its antiseptic action.

Imitates the oestrogen hormone and often useful with menstrual problems such as scanty periods, engorgement of breasts and gives rapid expulsion of afterbirth. Could well have some effect on conception difficulties.

Useful for wasp and insect bites, indeed, once reduced severe fevers like Malaria caused by parasites in the blood from mosquito bites.

May help to minimise uric acid in the blood and relieve gout as well as muscular pain generally. Stimulates blood flow and useful for deep muscle spasm.

EFFECT ON SKIN: A refreshing and tonic action benefits sluggish and congested skins and may also help to control acne.

BLENDS: Bergamot, Black Pepper, Clary Sage, Geranium, Hyssop, Lavender, Marjoram, Melissa, Neroli, Sandalwood, Verbena.

BAY

Plant/Part	:	Tree/Leaf
Latin Name	:	Laurus nobilis
Family	:	Lauraceae
Note	:	Top
Planet	:	Sun
Extraction	:	Distillation

AROMA: Sweet and spicy, a little like Cinnamon.

FEATURES: This sturdy evergreen tree grows to over thirty feet and is actually native to southern Europe. It's another variety 'Pimenta racemosa' which flavours West Indian Bay Rum. Our Bay tree has long lance-shaped leaves which are rather leathery and glossy and bear small creamy-yellow flowers and black berries. The oil is often obtained from Morocco and Spain.

HISTORY & MYTH: Extensively used by the ancient Egyptians and popular with the Romans who saw the Bay as a symbol of wisdom, protection and peace. Apollo, the god of healing was associated with the Bay tree. Its Latin derivative, 'Laudis', means 'to praise' hence the presentation of Laurel wreaths to victors at the Olympic Games. The idea of the 'Poet Laureate' descends from this practise.

A myth goes that pleasant and prophetic dreams occur if a Bay leaf is placed under the pillow. More practically, it has long been used in soups and sauces since it aids the digestion by increasing salivary secretion. Church floors in Greece are still strewn with Bay leaves perhaps due to their antiseptic quality. The durable wood has been used for making walking sticks. Sometimes referred to as 'Laurel'.

CHEMICAL CONSTITUENTS: Geraniol, Linalool, Terpineol (Alcohols), Cineole (Ketone), Eugenol (Phenol), Phellandrene, Pinene (Terpenes).

PROPERTIES: Analgesic, Antineuralgic, Antiseptic, Antispasmodic, Aperitif, Astringent, Cholagogue, Diuretic, Emmenagogue, Febrifuge, Hepatic, Insecticide, Parturient, Stimulant, Stomachic, Sudorific, Tonic.

PRECAUTIONS: The Romans liked nothing better than to soak in a bath sprinkled with Bay leaves. The essential oil however, may irritate the skin and possibly the mucous membranes so best used with caution or not at all. Pregnant women should stay clear of it.

MIND: Has a mildly narcotic and warming effect on the emotions.

BODY: Gives a pronounced action on the digestive system and could act as an appetite stimulant. Expels wind, settles stomach pain and has a tonic effect on the liver and kidneys. Promotes the flow of urine.

Rheumatic pain may be relieved by its application as well as general aches, pains and sprains, especially when combined with Rose and Juniper. Indicated particularly where there is a feeling of cold.

At the same time, it is said to bring down fever through its sweating action. Reputedly effective in infectious diseases and possibly helpful in cases of bronchitis.

Has a tonic action on the reproductive system, regulates scanty periods and speeds up delivery in childbirth.

May also help to ease ear infections thereby mitigating feelings of dizziness and restoring balance.

EFFECT ON SKIN: Has a reputation for being a good hair and scalp tonic, stimulating growth and clearing dandruff. It apparently helps to disperse blood in bruises, soothe inflammation and minimise scarring.

BLENDS: Cedarwood, Coriander, Eucalyptus, Ginger, Juniper, Lavender, Lemon, Marjoram, Orange, Rose, Rosemary, Thyme, Ylang Ylang.

BENZOIN

Plant/Part	:	Tree/Gum from trunk
Latin Name	:	Styrax benzoin
Family	:	Styraceae
Note	:	Base
Planet	:	Sun
Extraction	:	Solvent Extraction

AROMA: Sweet, like vanilla.

FEATURES: Java, Sumatra and Thailand gives us the Benzoin tree. Triangular wounds are cut into the bark from which the sap exudes – it does not occur naturally. The greyish brown, resinous lump is pressed into a solid mass and is not strictly an essential oil, more a resin. It is melted by heating over water before it can be used. Can be bought already dissolved in ethyl glycol.

HISTORY & MYTH: A scented gum, used in cosmetics for hundreds of years. The ancient civilisations thought it a grand remedy for driving away evil spirits and was often used in fumigations and incense. More recently it gained popularity as an ingredient of 'Friar's Balsam'. It was often referred to in old herbals as 'gum benzoin', 'balsam' or 'gum benjamin'. 'Virgin Milk', an old fashioned toilet water, included Benzoin as well as Lavender and Ethanol. It was supposed to make the skin 'clear and brilliant'. Nowadays used frequently as a fixative in perfumes.

CHEMICAL CONSTITUENTS: Benzoic, Cinnamic (Acids), Benzoic aldehyde, Vanillin (Aldehydes), Benzyl benzoate (Ester).

PROPERTIES: Antiseptic, Astringent, Carminative, Cephalic, Cordial, Deodorant, Diuretic, Expectorant, Sedative, Vulnerary.

PRECAUTIONS: Best avoided when concentration is needed – could have a drowsy effect.

MIND: A palliative for tension and stress since it has a calming effect on the nervous system. Brings comfort to the sad, lonely and depressed. Helps to let go of worries, instils confidence and eases exhausted emotional and psychic states.

BODY: Seems to have a rejuvenating effect on the body. It warms the heart and circulation and may ease general aches and pains as well as arthritis.

Has a good reputation for helping with respiratory disorders. It's a tonic to the lungs and has a beneficial action on bronchitis, asthma, coughs, colds, laryngitis and sore throats. Very effective on congested mucous membranes, expelling fluid waste.

Also helps with disorders of the urinary tract such as cystitis since it aids urine flow. A remedy for genital problems like leucorrhoea and may have a part to play with sexual difficulties, reputedly premature ejaculation.

Calming effect on the stomach, expels flatulence and strengthens the pancreas aiding digestion. Said to control blood sugar levels which could be helpful to sufferers of diabetes.

Apparently reduces mouth ulcers.

EFFECT ON SKIN: Sound remedy for cracked, dry skin, making it more elastic. Particularly useful for chapped hands and heels as well as chilblains and rashes. A good remedy for wounds and sores, valuable where there is redness, irritation and itching as in dermatitis.

BLENDS: Bergamot, Coriander, Cypress, Frankincense, Juniper, Lavender, Lemon, Myrrh, Orange, Petitgrain, Rose, Sandalwood.

BERGAMOT

Plant/Part	:	Tree/peel
Latin Name	:	Citrus bergamia
Family	:	Rutaceae
Note	:	Top
Planet	:	?
Extraction	:	Expression

AROMA: Light, delicate and refreshing. Something like orange and lemon with slight floral overtones.

FEATURES: Not to be confused with 'Monarda Didyma', a decorative flower also called Bergamot. Citrus Bergamia is a fifteen foot tree with long green leaves and white flowers. The fruit is pitted like a small orange although has a pear-like shape. Oil usually obtained from Italy and Morocco. The Bergamot tree, most delicate of all citrus plants, demands a special climate and soil.

HISTORY & MYTH: The oil takes its name from a small town in Italy where the tree was originally cultivated. However, legend has it that Christopher Columbus found the tree in the Canary Islands and introduced it into Spain and Italy. Records show its use in Florence since 1725 where it was popular in Italian folklore medicine but only recently exported.

A cheaper form of Bergamot oil is distilled from unripe fallen fruit and sometimes used to adulterate the more expensive oil. The leaves are occasionally distilled which gives us another form of Petitgrain. Bergamot imparts that unusual flavour to Earl Grey tea. Often used for its uplifting qualities in Aromatherapy and may be a first choice for depressive states. Probably one of the most common ingredients of all perfumes, especially Eau de Cologne.

CHEMICAL CONSTITUENTS: Linalool, Nerol, Terpineol (Alcohols), Linalyl acetate (Ester), Bergaptene (Lactone), Dipentene, Limonene (Terpenes).

PROPERTIES: Analgesic, Antidepressant, Antiseptic, Antispasmodic, Carminative, Cicatrisant, Cordial, Deodorant, Digestive, Expectorant, Febrifuge, Insecticide, Sedative, Stomachic, Tonic, Vermifuge, Vulnerary.

PRECAUTIONS: Strong sunlight to be avoided after use as it increases photosensitivity of the skin. This is due to the chemical Bergaptene which will help with tanning but not protect from burning. May also irritate sensitive skin.

MIND: Its sedative yet uplifting character is excellent for anxiety, depression and nervous tension. A combined cooling and refreshing quality seems to allay anger and frustration probably by decreasing action of the Sympathetic Nervous System.

BODY: A valuable antiseptic for the urinary tract and effective with infection and inflammation, chiefly cystitis.

Also works well on the digestive tract and relieves conditions such as painful digestion, dyspepsia, flatulence, colic, indigestion and loss of appetite. An excellent intestinal antiseptic, casts out intestinal parasites and diminishes gall stones apparently. May be useful to anorexia sufferers by regulating appetite.

Also helpful with infections of the respiratory system which may include breathing difficulties as well as tonsillitis, bronchitis and tuberculosis. Often effective on cold sores, chicken pox and shingles.

Could have a tonic action on the uterus and was once used to heal sexually transmitted diseases.

Excellent insect repellent and keeps pets away from plants.

EFFECT ON SKIN: Its antiseptic and healing action seems to benefit oily skin conditions, especially when linked to stress. These may include eczema, psoriasis, acne, scabies, varicose ulcers, wounds, herpes, seborrhoea of the skin and scalp. Excellent for skin sores in combination with Eucalyptus.

BLENDS: Chamomile, Coriander, Cypress, Eucalyptus, Geranium, Juniper, Jasmine, Lavender, Lemon, Marjoram, Neroli, Palmarosa, Patchouli, Ylang Ylang.

BIRCH

Plant/Part	:	Tree/Bark/Twigs
Latin Name	:	Betula alleghaniensis (yellow)
		Betula pendula (Silver)
		Betula lenta (Cherry)
Family	:	Betulaceae
Note	:	Top
Planet	:	Venus or Mercury
Extraction	:	Maceration & Distillation

AROMA: A rather antiseptic though refreshing aroma.

FEATURES: A very large woodland tree, distinguished by the catkins it bears. Some of the 100 different varieties can reach to about eighty feet and often have slim branches pointing downwards with serrated oval leaves. B. alleghaniensis originally comes from the United States, B. pendula and B. lenta from USSR, Holland and Germany. B. lenta is the smallest variety and also known as Sweet Birch. Prior to distillation the bark of B. lenta has to be macerated in lukewarm water to free the essential oil.

HISTORY & MYTH: Appears to have a connection with warding off evil spirits though more practically, the juice of the leaves once made an excellent gargle for mouth sores. Throughout the centuries, the sap has been used in making medicinal wine and the leaves were made into a diuretic tea. Also an ingredient of skin lotions and liniments possibly due to its astringent properties and has latterly been used in perfumes.

Russia once supplied Birch Tar Oil which was employed in the manufacture of leather and soaps though it was also helpful for rheumatic joints, gout and skin infections. B. Alba was a hair tonic ingredient called 'Birkenwasser' popular in Germany. Its main chemical ingredient, Methyl Salicylate, gives us aspirin indicating pain relieving properties. Imparts a 'leathery' odour to mens toiletries though probably more popular in France. The strong timber has often been used in making furniture, house and farm implements. Often seen as a decorative street tree.

CHEMICAL CONSTITUENTS: Salicylic (Acid), Methyl salicylate (Ester), Betulene, Betulenol (Sesquiterpenes).

PROPERTIES: Analgesic, Antiseptic, Astringent, Depurative, Disinfectant, Diuretic, Insecticide, Tonic.

PRECAUTIONS: A powerful oil and could irritate sensitive skin. Best used with caution or not at all.

MIND: Has an invigorating, even rousing effect on the spirits.

BODY: A generally purifying oil: cleanses the blood, stimulates the sweat glands aiding the body in releasing harmful toxins. A lymphatic cleanser and helps keep infection at bay.

It increases the flow of urine, eliminating organic wastes and eases painful cystitis. Also reputedly clears albuminuria – a protein in the urine. Dissolves stones in the bladder and kidneys. Effective against renal oedema, producing a general tonic action on the kidneys.

Its diuretic properties could also help with obesity, cellulitis and dropsy.

Eliminates accumulation of uric acid in the joints and could be good for rheumatism, arthritis and muscle pain generally. Said to have a really strong pain-killing action.

EFFECT ON SKIN: Possibly has an effective healing action on chronic skin ailments such as eczema, psoriasis, acne and skin ulcers.

BLENDS: Cardamom, Chamomile, Frankincense, Ginger, Lavender, Lemon, Orange, Tagetes, Cajeput, Thyme.

BLACK PEPPER

Plant/Part	:	Shrub/Fruit
Latin Name	:	Piper nigrum
Family	:	Piperaceae
Note	:	Middle
Planet	:	Mars
Extraction	:	Distillation

AROMA: Very sharp and spicy.

FEATURES: Dark green leaves, white flowers and red fruits adorn this climbing vine-like shrub. Originally a forest plant, Black Pepper thrives best in the shade. It naturally grows to over twenty feet often needing support, however, these days it is cultivated to just twelve feet. The oil is derived from Black Pepper rather than White, since it is more aromatic and contains greater amounts of oil. Cultivated in the East, the oil is mainly obtained from Singapore, India and Malaysia.

HISTORY & MYTH: A very old and highly revered spice, used in India over 4,000 years ago, mainly for urinary and liver disorders and probably for cholera and dysentery as well. The root word comes originally from the Sanskrit 'pippali', changing to the Latin 'piper'.

So popular with the Romans that taxes were paid with it instead of coins. The Greeks used it extensively for combating fever and the Turks levelled a high tax on caravans carrying Pepper through its lands. During the Middle Ages the Pepper trade was very important between India and Europe often resulting in naval wars between the Portuguese, French and Dutch. The Portuguese had the monopoly until 19th century. During its chequered history, Black Pepper has been used to treat gonorrhoea and urethritis.

CHEMICAL CONSTITUENTS: Eugenol, Myristicin, Safrole (Phenol), Bisabolene, Camphene, Farnesene, Limonene, Myrcene, Phellandrene, Pinene, Sabinene, Selinene, Thujene (Terpenes), Caryophyllene (Sesquiterpene).

PROPERTIES: Analgesic, Antiemetic, Antiseptic, Antispasmodic, Aphrodisiac, Cardiac, Carminative, Detoxicant, Digestive, Diuretic, Febrifuge, Laxative, Rubefacient, Stimulant, Stomachic, Tonic.

PRECAUTIONS: Too much too often may over stimulate the kidneys. Possibility of skin irritation.

MIND: Very stimulating, strengthens the nerves and mind. Gives stamina where there is frustration, warms the heart where there is indifference.

BODY: Gives tone to skeletal muscles. Dilation of local blood vessels makes it useful for muscular aches and pains, tired and aching limbs and muscular stiffness. Good oil to use before excessive exertion like sport. Also helpful with rheumatoid arthritis and temporary paralysis of the limbs.

Fortifying effect on the stomach, increases flow of saliva and stimulates appetite. Expels wind, quells vomiting and encourages peristalsis. Useful in bowel problems generally as it restores tone to colon muscles. Said to be an antidote for fish and mushroom poisoning. Promotes urine and stimulates the kidneys.

Banishes excess fat! Perhaps by aiding digestion of protein, such as rich meats. Generally expels toxins.

Stimulates the circulation and may be helpful with anaemia since it reputedly aids the formation of new blood cells.

Has a beneficial effect on respiratory illnesses particularly where there is a feeling of cold. Yet can bring down high temperatures in very small amounts.

EFFECT ON SKIN: Helpful with bruises.

BLENDS: Basil, Bergamot, Cypress, Frankincense, Geranium, Grapefruit, Lemon, Palmarosa, Rosemary, Sandalwood, Ylang Ylang.

CAJUPUT

Plant/Part	:	Tree/Leaves and twigs
Latin Name	:	Melaleuca leucadendron
Family	:	Myrtaceae
Note	:	Top
Planet	:	?
Extraction	:	Distillation

AROMA: Sweet, herbaceous and rather penetrating.

FEATURES: This vigorous tree, originally from the coastal plains of Malaya, reaches to about forty five feet. It is also found in the Philippines, the Moluccas and Australia and has a whitish bark with a crooked trunk. It tends to crowd out other trees and cultivation is minimal since spontaneous regrowth occurs after destruction. Caju-pute in Malay means white tree and often referred to as White Tea Tree.

HISTORY & MYTH: Cajuput has a myriad of uses in the East finding its way into the cooking pot as well as being an ingredient of cosmetics and perfumes. Revered for its antiseptic properties, it has long been a popular household medication in Malaya, India and China. Looked upon as a panacea against stomach troubles and skin diseases, it was also the traditional remedy for rheumatism and cholera. Often used as a room spray to ward off insects and bed bugs. In ancient India it was known as Kayaputi.

CONSTITUENTS: Terpineol (Alcohol), Benzaldehyde (Aldehyde), Cineole (Ketone), Dipentene, Limonene, Pinene (Terpenes).

PROPERTIES: Analgesic, Antidontalgic, Antineuralgic, Antirheumatic, Antiseptic, Antispasmodic, Balsamic, Cicatrisant, Decongestant, Expectorant, Febrifuge, Insecticide, Pectoral, Stimulant, Sudorific, Vermifuge.

PRECAUTIONS: A powerful oil and should be used with caution. Could in some cases irritate the skin and mucous membranes.

MIND: Rather stimulating, clears thought, awakens sluggish feelings and helps put the body and mind back into balance.

BODY: Excellent antiseptic for the respiratory tract. Its sudorific properties help to minimise feverish colds by exerting a cooling influence. A drop in the bath promotes sweating, releasing 'flu toxins and is also effective in inhalations. Particularly beneficial at the start of infections such as in colds, pharyngitis, laryngitis and bronchitis. Said to ease chronic pulmonary disease generally and may be helpful for asthma.

Soothes colic and inflammation of the intestines such as enteritis, dysentery, gastric spasm, nervous vomiting and intestinal parasites.

Also has an antiseptic effect on the urinary system and could help with cystitis and urethritis.

Its pain relieving properties may be good for neuralgia, headaches, toothache (almost as effective as Clove apparently!), earache, gout, chronic rheumatism, muscle stiffness and general aches and pains.

Also said to imitate the hormone oestrogen and may alleviate menopausal problems and settle period pains.

Renowned as an antidote against insect bites and headlice. Fleas and lice apparently make a hasty exit when pets are rubbed down with this oil.

EFFECT ON SKIN: Said to be beneficial for chronic skin conditions such as acne and psoriasis.

BLENDS: Angelica, Bergamot, Birch, Cardamom, Clove, Geranium, Immortelle, Lavender, Myrtle, Niaouli, Nutmeg, Rose, Rosewood, Thyme.

CAMPHOR

Plant/Part	:	Tree/Wood
Latin Name	:	Cinnamomum camphora
Family	:	Lauraceae
Note	:	Base
Planet	:	?
Extraction	:	Distillation

AROMA: Fresh, clean and very piercing.

FEATURES: Grown in the East principally Borneo, China, Sri Lanka, Madagascar and Sumatra. A very hardy, evergreen tree reaching to around a hundred feet. White flowers and red berries adorn the small and slightly serrated leaves. This long lived tree – often up to a thousand years – is not touched until it is about fifty years old. Camphor is found in every part of the tree, though the colourless, crystalline mass takes many years to form. Oil from the Borneocamphor tree 'Dryobalanops camphora' native to Sumatra and from the Dipterocarpaceae family, is often preferred in Aromatherapy as it is not so harsh.

HISTORY & MYTH: Some Far Eastern civilisations saw it as a plant sacred to the gods and it was often used for ceremonial purposes. Battling heroes were crowned with the leaves though its use in embalming was widespread too. The strong aroma appealed to the Chinese who imported it from Vietnam to build their ships and temples. Persia – now Iran – once considered it a powerful remedy against the Plague. Their King Chrosroes 11, esteemed it highly enough to preserve it among the treasures of his palace in Babylon. Archaeologists, during a dig in Italy, found organic matter perfectly preserved in a jar of Borneo. It has long been an important essential oil used world wide for aromatics and insecticides.

CONSTITUENTS: Camphor: Camphor (Ketone), Safrole (Phenol), Borneol (Alcohol), Camphene (Terpene). **Borneo:** Borneol (Alcohol), Pinene, Camphene, Dipentene (Terpenes).

PROPERTIES: Analgesic, Antidepressant, Antiseptic, Antispasmodic, Cardiac, Carminative, Diuretic, Febrifuge, Hypertensive, Insecticide, Laxative, Rubefacient, Stimulant, Sudorific, Vermifuge, Vulnerary.

PRECAUTIONS: A powerful oil, very stimulating and overdosing could cause convulsions and vomiting. Should be avoided in pregnancy and people suffering from epilepsy and asthma. White Camphor oil is said to be less toxic than the yellow and brown variety which contain large amounts of Safrole. Japanese Camphor contains Ketones.

MIND: A balancing oil despite its primary stimulating nature. Sedates nervy types particularly when associated with depression yet rouses apathy – could be helpful in convalescence. Apparently has a beneficial effect on psychosomatic or nervous diseases.

BODY: Stimulates the heart, respiration and circulation. It raises low blood pressure. Clears congested lungs, eases breathing and often used as an inhalant.

Seems to be helpful to any condition where there is a feeling of cold from the common bug to pneumonia though its balancing action can help with inflammation. It puts the body in balance, warms and cools where necessary.

Effect on digestion is calming; good for constipation and diarrhoea. Also helpful with gastro enteritis. Works on the urinary system (allows urination) and relieves irritation of the sexual organs.

May be helpful with stiff muscles therefore of particular use in sport though often seen as a palliative for rheumatic aches and pains as well.

In the past it was found to be useful for such serious diseases as cholera, pneumonia and tuberculosis. Good for keeping infection down generally.

EFFECT ON SKIN: Action on the skin is cooling and therefore reduces inflammatory conditions. Oily skins seem to benefit most and could help in cases of acne, burns and ulcers. Cold compresses for bruises and sprains are usually effective.

BLENDS: Basil, Cajuput, Chamomile, Lavender, Melissa.

CARAWAY

Plant/Part	:	Herb/Seeds
Latin Name	:	Carum carvi
Family	:	Umbelliferae
Note	:	Top
Planet	:	Mercuty
Extraction	:	Distillation

AROMA: Sweet, sharp and slightly peppery.

FEATURES: Cultivated in Northern Europe, Africa and Russia, though the plant actually originates from Caria, a country of Asia-Minor. The fruit closely resembles Cumin and Fennel and the plant grows to about two feet. It has soft fern-like leaves and small, curved brown fruits with tufted pink/white flowers.

HISTORY & MYTH: Sometimes known as 'Meadow Cumin', it is a very old spice, dating back to the Stone-age. The Egyptians flavoured their food with it and traces of Caraway have been found in their burial places. The Romans used it in breadmaking possibly because of its carminative properties and was often eaten at the end of meals.

Also celebrated in Arabia from where the name 'Karawya' comes. Seems to have gained a reputation for sharpening the eyesight and sweetening the breath as well as guarding against loss of loved ones! In India it was used in the manufacture of soap. A popular herb throughout the middle ages especially in German and Austrian cooking. An ingredient of 'Kummel' liqueur. Prince Albert, Queen Victoria's consort, apparently introduced it to England.

CHEMICAL CONSTITUENTS: Acetaldehyde, Cuminic aldehyde, Furfurol (Aldehyde), Carvone (Ketone), Limonene (Terpenes).

PROPERTIES: Antiseptic, Antispasmodic, Aperitif, Astringent, Cardiac, Carminative, Depurative, Digestive, Disinfectant, Diuretic, Emmenagogue, Expectorant, Galactagogue, Parasiticide, Stimulant, Vermifuge.

PRECAUTIONS: A potent oil and may irritate sensitive skin. Debatable whether should be used in massage.

MIND: Warming to the emotions, tonic to the nerves and helps to ease mental strain and fatigue. Seems to replenish lost energy.

BODY: Has a calming effect on stomach disorders particularly pain, gastric spasm and flatulence. Settles the digestion and stimulates appetite. Gives relief from diarrhoea and general bowel complaints. Its reputation as a breath sweetener may be well founded since it appears to have some effect on gastric fermentations.

Seems to have a beneficial action on urinary problems by increasing the urine and flushing out toxins. May be a tonic to the liver easing hepatitis.

Its expectorant properties may help with bronchitis and bronchial asthma. Also helpful to other throat and lung problems like laryngitis and aerophagy (swallowing gulps of air).

Increases milk in nursing mothers and may be a general tonic to the glandular system. Apparently helpful with period pains.

Good for earache and diminishes vertigo. It also has a stimulating effect on the circulation. Overall, seems to get the body going again.

EFFECT ON SKIN: An effective tissue regenerator and particularly helpful for oily skin conditions. Has been known to disperse bruises, reduce boils and clean infected wounds. Other benefits include relief from itchy skin, acne, scalp problems and scabies. If that wasn't enough, was once used to liven up pale complexions too.

BLENDS: Basil, Bay, Benzoin, Cardamom, Chamomile, Coriander, Elemi, Frankincense, Galbanum, Geranium, Ginger, Lavender, Orange, Rosewood.

CARDAMOM

Plant/Part	:	Reed/Seeds
Latin Name	:	Elettaria cardamomum
Family	:	Zingiberaceae
Note	:	Top
Planet	:	?
Extraction	:	Distillation

AROMA: Sweet and spicy almost like bitter-lemons.

FEATURES: Grows wild and under cultivation in India, Ceylon and Indo-China though the oil is obtained from South America and France. It is a leafy stemmed shrub reaching up to eighteen feet with very long leaves and pale yellow flowers sporting a mauve tip. The oblong, grey fruits contain many seeds and are gathered just before they are ripe.

HISTORY & MYTH: Long used as a condiment and medicine in India and was generally thought to have a good effect on the digestive system, easing piles and jaundice as well as urinary complaints. The Egyptians thought it rather nice to use in perfumes and incense and they also chewed the seeds to keep their teeth white. These days however, Cardamom is often ground with their coffee.

The Romans used it to settle their stomachs after gastronomical feasts and the Arabs agreed that it had sound digestive properties. They also thought it was an effective aphrodisiac. Often employed in Eastern European cooking as it apparently disguises the smell of garlic. It has also enjoyed popular use as an ingredient in some eau-de-colognes. The essential oil is said to have been distilled for the first time around the year 1544 after discovery by the Portuguese.

CHEMICAL CONSTITUENTS: Terpineol (Alcohol), Cineole (Ketone), Limonene, Sabinene, Terpinene (Terpenes).

PROPERTIES: Antiseptic, Antispasmodic, Aperitif, Aphrodisiac, Carminative, Cephalic, Digestive, Diuretic, Sialagogue, Stimulant, Stomachic, Tonic.

PRECAUTIONS: Sensitive skins beware – could cause allergy.

MIND: Warming to the senses particularly where there is a feeling of weakness and fatigue. Uplifting, refreshing and invigorating, clearing confusion perhaps.

BODY: Particularly helpful with digestive problems especially of nervous origin. Can work as a laxative and deals with colic, wind, dyspepsia (discomfort in upper digestive tract) and pyrosis (a burning sensation in the stomach). Eases feelings of nausea and effective against bad breath as it deals with gastric fermentation. Encourages flow of saliva and stimulates loss of appetite.

May act on bile production since it reputedly diminishes bodily fats. Its diuretic action could be useful when difficulty exists in passing urine.

Its reputation as an aphrodisiac may perhaps be due to its tonic effect on the body possibly dealing with low sexual response. Certainly has been a remedy for impotence for some time. Also appears to ease feelings of irritation during pre menstrual tension as well as headaches.

Also works well on the respiratory system, eases coughs and warms the body when feeling cold.

EFFECT ON SKIN: ?

BLENDS: Coriander, Frankincense, Galbanum, Geranium, Juniper, Lemon, Myrtle, Pine, Rosewood, Verbena.

CARROT SEED

Plant/Part	:	Herb/Seed
Latin Name	:	Daucus carota
Family	:	Umbelliferae
Note	:	Middle
Planet	:	Mercury
Extraction	:	Distillation

AROMA: Slightly sweet and dry.

FEATURES: The essential oil is obtained mainly from the wild carrot though the domestic variety gets a look in too. Stalks and leaves of both varieties are similar though the wild type has a slightly rougher texture and the root is not edible. White flowers with purple centres adorn the stalks. The whole plant yields an essential oil which usually hails from Europe, though some is also obtained from Egypt and India.

HISTORY & MYTH: The Carrot was of great medicinal value in the ancient world and the name stems from the Greek 'Carotos'. Recognised for its carminative and hepatic properties, it has grown in popularity since the 16th century. It also gained a reputation for dealing with skin diseases.

These days it is apparently used on cancer patients especially those with stomach and throat problems. It may have an effect on skin cancers too, since it contains carotene (converts to Vitamin A), responsible for keeping skin, hair, teeth and gums healthy. The carrot has long been associated with good eyesight as well as shortening the duration of illness. The oil is a popular ingredient for flavouring food substitutes, alcoholic liqueurs and some perfume compositions.

CHEMICAL CONSTITUENTS: Acetic (Acid), Carotol (Alcohol), Asarone (Phenol), Bisabolene, Limonene, Pinene (Terpenes).

PROPERTIES: Carminative, Cytophylactic, Depurative, Diuretic, Emmenagogue, Hepatic, Stimulant, Tonic, Vermifuge.

PRECAUTIONS: Probably best avoided in pregnancy.

MIND: A cleansing effect on the mind could relieve feelings of stress and exhaustion.

BODY: An excellent purifier of the body, mainly due to its detoxifying effect on the liver. Can possibly help with jaundice as well as other liver problems. Reputedly expels kidney stones and eases hepatitis.

Also cleanses the bowels, controls flatulence and stems diarrhoea. May relieve painful stomach ulcers. Releases fluid retention and eases cystitis. Seems to relieve gout as well.

By increasing red blood corpuscles it boosts the general action of the organs improving energy output. Possibly helpful with anaemia too and its attendant symptoms of weakness and exhaustion.

Seems to work well with respiratory problems such as influenza and bronchitis since it strengthens the mucous membranes of the nose, throat and lungs. Also said to ease coughs and chilblains.

Reputedly helpful to the reproductive system by its tonic action on the hormones. Its regulation of the menstrual cycle could assist in cases of infertility, aiding conception.

EFFECT ON SKIN: Improves the complexion due to its strengthening effect on red blood cells, adding tone and elasticity to the skin. Gives a more 'youthful' appearance apparently and said to remove 'age' spots. A panacea for premature ageing and keeping wrinkles at bay – perhaps due to its formative action on epidermal cells. This may also help scarring. Also said to alleviate other problems such as weeping sores and ulcers, vitiligo (lack of pigment), pruritus, boils, carbuncles, eczema, psoriasis. Generally healing to inflamed wounds as well as dry and hard skin, callouses and corns.

BLENDS: Bergamot, Juniper, Lavender, Lemon, Lime, Melissa, Neroli, Orange, Petitgrain, Rosemary, Verbena.

CEDARWOOD

Plant/Part	:	Tree/Wood
Latin Name	:	Juniperus virginiana (Red) Cedrus atlantica (White)
Family	:	Cupressaceae/Pinaceae
Note	:	Base
Planet	:	Sun
Extraction	:	Distillation

AROMA: Woody, reminiscent of Sandalwood but slightly 'dryer'.

FEATURES: Juniperus Virginiana, a large red cedar, is from North America though another species, the Cedrus Atlantica, comes from Morocco. Both are said to produce oil which is similar in therapeutic action.

HISTORY & MYTH: Cedar is a Semitic word meaning the power of spiritual strength and represents a symbol of constant faith. One of the oldest aromatics used as temple incense, which may have added to its mystical image. The ancient Egyptians used the oil extensively, particularly in mummification. Also the wood was a popular medium for making sarcophagi as well as the tall masts in Egyptian ships. Once employed for large buildings like temples but now used for small items, such as boxes, pencils etc as the wood tends to warp. The species used in antiquity (Cedrus Libani), related to C. Atlantica, is now very scarce due to overuse.

The oil was also an Eastern remedy for the treatment of gonorrhoea when Sandalwood was unavailable. In North America, it was used for bronchitis, tuberculosis and skin diseases. 'Mithvidat' – a centuries-old antidote against poisons included Cedarwood as one of its ingredients. Nowadays, Cedarwood is a popular fixative in perfumes.

CHEMICAL CONSTITUENTS: Cedrol (Alcohol), Cadinene, Cedrene, Cedrenol (Sesquiterpenes).

PROPERTIES: Antiseptic, Astringent, Diuretic, Emollient, Expectorant, Fungicide, Insecticide, Sedative, Tonic.

PRECAUTIONS: High concentrations may possibly irritate the skin. Best avoided in pregnancy.

MIND: Nervous tension and anxious states benefit greatly by its calming and soothing action. This makes it a valuable aid to meditation though its reputation for steering strayed individuals back on the path needs to be tested.

BODY: Tends to be useful for long standing complaints rather than acute ones. A combined tonic action on the glandular and nervous system helps put the body back into balance thereby regulating homeostasis.

Its main effect however, probably due to its expectorant properties, is on the respiratory tract and may help ease conditions such as bronchitis, coughs and catarrh. Excess phlegm is curbed through Cedarwood's 'drying' effect.

Also of importance to the genito-urinary tract reducing problems such as cystitis particularly where there is burning pain. Has a tonic effect on the kidneys.

Could relieve some painful cases of chronic rheumatism and arthritis.

EFFECT ON SKIN: Its astringent and antiseptic properties are of greatest benefit to oily skin conditions – could help acne. Also helps to clear scabs and pus and chronic conditions such as dermatitis and psoriasis. A good hair tonic and could be effective against seborrhoea of the scalp, dandruff and alopecia. Skin softening properties are enhanced apparently when mixed with Cypress and Frankincense.

BLENDS: Benzoin, Bergamot, Cinnamon, Cypress, Frankincense, Jasmine, Juniper, Lavender, Lemon, Linden Blossom, Neroli, Rose, Rosemary.

CELERY

Plant/Part	:	Herb/Seeds
Latin Name	:	Apium graveolens
Family	:	Umbelliferae
Note	:	Middle
Planet	:	Mercury
Extraction	:	Distillation

AROMA: Fresh and warm with a hint of spice.

FEATURES: A native of Eurasia, likes to grow in moist ground near the sea. The stem is smooth, about two feet high with whitish flowers and delicate light green leaves. The tiny brown seeds are crushed immediately before distillation. Oil often obtained from India and France.

HISTORY & MYTH: Apium comes from the Celtic 'apon' which means water and the Latin Graveolens implies gravity. A funereal association with Celery amongst the ancient Egyptians and Romans inclined them to see it as a symbol of grief and death. However, the Egyptians practical as ever, also used Celery to relieve swollen limbs.

In latter times, the Celery found growing around the salt marches in southern Europe, was further cultivated by the Italians during the 17th century. Several varieties have been developed from the original. Occasionally called 'scented smallage', indicating that all parts play an aromatic role in cooking and often used in soups and salads since it is rich in minerals and helpful in salt reduced diets. Culpeper maintained that the herb 'cleared female obstructions' which indicates a positive effect on the reproductive system. Has the distinction in being used as bird seed as well as nerve tonics and food flavourings.

CHEMICAL CONSTITUENTS: Sedanonic anhydride (Acid), Sedanolide (Lactone), Limonene, Selinene (Terpenes).

PROPERTIES: Antiphlogistic, Antirheumatic, Aphrodisiac, Carminative, Diuretic, Hypotensive, Sedative, Tonic.

PRECAUTIONS: ?

MIND: A sedative and tonic effect on the Central Nervous System is useful for nervous disorders, resulting in a feeling of joy – hopefully!

BODY: Its pronounced diuretic properties could help with weight problems exacerbated by water retention and cellulite. It also cleanses the bladder, liver and spleen. Seems to be effective in clearing the body of toxins by purifying the blood.

Widely used to dissolve accumulated uric acid in the joints, so may be useful in rheumatism, arthritis and gout.

Helpful to the digestive tract generally due to its carminative properties. Particularly useful in expelling wind and easing that bloated feeling.

Believed to assist in minimising sexual problems possibly because of its effect on anxiety and nervousness. Its rather earthy yet euphoric nature could instill a slightly intoxicating feeling. Could be therefore, that its reputation as an aphrodisiac is not unfounded! It is also said to bring down high blood pressure which may restore libido to those with heart problems.

Its antiphlogistic properties cools fevers generally and may have some effect on bronchitis.

EFFECT ON SKIN: Decreases puffiness and redness which may be symptoms of a water-logged skin.

BLENDS: Angelica, Basil, Cajuput, Chamomile, Grapefruit, Guaiacwood, Lemon, Orange, Palmarosa, Rosemary, Verbena.

CHAMOMILE

Plant/Part	:	Herb/dried flowers
Latin Name	:	Anthemis nobilis (Roman Chamomile) Matricaria chamomilia (German Chamomile)
Family	:	Compositae
Note	:	Middle
Planet	:	Sun
Extraction	:	Distillation

AROMA: A fruity, apple-like fragrance.

FEATURES: Indigenous to Britain and cultivated in Germany, France and Morocco. Both Roman and German Chamomile share many features; about 12 inches high with white flowers, yellow centre and slightly furry leaves. German Chamomile is a little smaller. Essential oil from both types contain Azuline (a powerful anti-inflammatory agent) not actually present in the plant but formed in the oil. German Chamomile contains a little more and is a deep blue colour – sometimes known as 'Hungarian Chamomile' – just to confuse the issue.

HISTORY & MYTH: According to Culpeper, the Egyptians dedicated this herb to the Sun since it cured fevers (heat). Other sources say it is a Moon herb because it has a cooling effect. Certainly the Egyptian priests recognised its soothing properties where nervous complaints were concerned. It has come down in history as the plants' physician because it cures other shrubs when planted nearby.

The name is derived from the Greek meaning 'ground apple' and the Latin 'nobilis' refers to noble flowers. Used extensively in shampoos throughout the ages particularly to highlight and condition fair hair. These days it is often employed in cosmetics and perfumes. Chamomile tea has been a popular aid to digestion as well as promoting sound sleep. Also thought to help jaundice and liver problems – perhaps that is why it is sometimes added to liqueurs!

CHEMICAL CONSTITUENTS: Anthemis Nobilis: Angelic, Methacrylic, Tiglic (Acid), Azuline (Sesquiterpene), Matricaria Chamomila: Cuminic (Aldehyde), Azuline (Sesquiterpene).

PROPERTIES: Analgesic, Antiallergenic, Anticonvulsive, Antidepressant, Antiemetic, Antiphlogistic, Antipruritic, Antirheumatic, Antiseptic, Antispasmodic, Carminative, Cholagogue, Cicatrisant, Digestive, Diuretic, Emollient, Emmenagogue, Febrifuge, Hepatic, Nervine, Sedative, Splenetic, Stomachic, Sudorific, Tonic, Vermifuge, Vulnerary.

PRECAUTIONS: An emmenagogue, so should be avoided in the early months of pregnancy.

MIND: A very soothing oil easing anxiety, tension, anger and fear. Promotes relaxation, gives patience, peace and allays worries. Calms the mind and often helpful with insomnia.

BODY: Its analgesic action eases dull muscular pain particularly when connected to nervous conditions. Low back pain seems to respond well. In the same way useful for headaches, neuralgia, toothache and earache.

Useful with menstrual problems since helps to regulate the menstrual cycle and eases period pain. Seems to be a popular choice for calming irritable effects of pre menstrual tension and the menopause.

Soothes the stomach and often relieves gastritis, diarrhoea, colitis, peptic ulcers, vomiting, wind, inflammation of the bowels – may be useful for irritable bowel syndrome. Also said to be helpful with liver problems, jaundice as well as disorders of the genito-urinary tract.

Indicated for use with repeated infections since stimulates production of white corpuscles which help to fight bacteria and fortify the defence system. Could be effective against anaemia.

EFFECT ON SKIN: Soothes burns, blisters, inflamed wounds, ulcers and boils. Could be helpful with dermatitis, acne, herpes, psoriasis, hypersensitive skins as well as allergic conditions generally. Smooths out broken capillaries, improving elasticity. Good for dry and itchy skin, eases puffiness and strengthens the tissues. An excellent skin cleanser.

BLENDS: Angelica, Benzoin, Bergamot, Geranium, Jasmine, Lavender, Lemon, Marjoram, Neroli, Palmarosa, Patchouli, Rose, Ylang Ylang.

CINNAMON

Plant/Part	:	Tree/Bud/Bark/Leaf
Latin Name	:	Cinnamomum zeylanicum
Family	:	Lauraceae
Note	:	Base
Planet	:	Mercury or Sun
Extraction	:	Distillation

AROMA: Spicy, sharp, sweet and musky.

FEATURES: This exotic rust coloured tree, which remains in full bloom all the year round, is native to Indonesia, though cultivated in Sri Lanka by the Dutch in the 18th century. It has pale brown, thick quills rolled inside one another and though naturally reaches to about thirty three feet is kept down to six feet for commercial reasons. Also found in the East Indies, Java and Madagascar.

HISTORY & MYTH: A very old spice, once regarded as a precious substance particularly for use as temple incense. Indeed, the mythical Phoenix collected Cinnamon as well as Myrrh and Spikenard for use in the magic fire in which it was reborn. The Egyptians thought it a good oil for the feet as well as an excellent remedy for excessive bile. Around 4,000 years ago, it was an important trade item between India, China and Egypt.

The Chinese used it for excessive gas and to normalise temperature in the liver. The Greeks came to value it for its stomachic and antiseptic properties and the Romans included it in their famous perfume 'Susinum'. Used in Europe since about 9th century as an ingredient of mulled wine and love potions, it was also given as a sedative to mothers during childbirth. When England took over Sri Lanka in the late 18th century the Cinnamon industry became a monopoly of the important East India Company.

CHEMICAL CONSTITUENTS: Linalool (Alcohol), Benzaldehyde, Cinnamic, Furfurol (Aldehyde), Eugenol, Safrole (Phenols), Cymene, Dipentene, Phellandrene, Pinene (Terpenes).

PROPERTIES: Anaesthetic, Antidontalgic, Antiseptic, Antiputrefactive, Antispasmodic, Aphrodisiac, Astringent, Cardiac, Carminative, Emmenagogue, Escharotic, Haemostatic, Insecticide, Parasiticide, Sialogogue, Stimulant, Stomachic, Vermifuge.

PRECAUTIONS: Cinnamon Leaf essential oil is often preferred over Cinnamon Bark or Bud as the latter two may in some cases cause a severe skin reaction, having a large proportion of Cinnamic Aldehyde often the cause of skin sensitisation. Nevertheless, Cinnamon Leaf is a very powerful oil and should be used with care. Best avoided in pregnancy as it could be abortifacient. High dosage could cause convulsions.

MIND: Excellent for exhausted states and feelings of weakness and depression.

BODY: A very strong antiseptic and has a tonic effect on the respiratory tract, eases colds through its very warming action by slightly raising body temperature, indicated for influenza. Generally restores heat to the body. Eases breathing difficulties and restores the senses during fainting fits. Has an excellent reputation for resisting viral infections and contagious diseases.

Seems to have a spurring action on bodily fluids since it stimulates tears, saliva and mucous.

A palliative for intestinal infections. Calms spasm of the digestive tract, asthenia (loss of tone), dyspepsia, colitis, flatulence, gastralgia, diarrhoea, nausea and vomiting. Stimulates secretion of gastric juices. In the past used for serious diseases such as cholera and typhoid.

A strong stimulant of the glandular system indicates its use in easing period pain as well as regulating scanty menstruation and leucorrhoea. Its aphrodisiac properties reputedly effective in cases of impotence.

Has a tonic effect on the whole body and particularly on the circulatory system. May also ease muscular spasm and painful rheumatic joints.

Seems to take the sting out of insect bites.

EFFECT ON SKIN: Has a mildly astringent effect on the skin tightening loose tissues and apparently effective in clearing warts.

BLENDS: Benzoin, Cardamom, Clove, Coriander, Frankincense, Galbanum, Ginger, Grapefruit, Lavender, Orange, Pine, Rosemary, Thyme.

CITRONELLA

Plant/Part	:	Grass/Cut grass
Latin Name	:	Cymbopogon nardus
Family	:	Graminae
Note	:	Top
Planet	:	?
Extraction	:	Distillation

AROMA: Slightly sweet and lemony.

FEATURES: A hardy grass, grown mainly in Sri Lanka and Java though also found in Burma, Madagascar, Guatemala and South America. It was formerly known as Andropogon Nardus. The plant reaches to about three feet and has long slender leaves which flower when left in their natural state. Preference is given to distillation of the dried grass rather than the fresh material which would require too much fuel and is said to yield an oil of less agreeable odour.

HISTORY & MYTH: Originally grown in Sri Lanka and came into vogue in the last century. The first shipment of oil to Europe was known as 'Oleum siree'. Sri Lanka was the main importer until 1890, when Java started producing the oil, apparently of superior quality. It contained greater quantities of Geraniol (Alcohol) and has a stronger odour. The Sri Lankan oil used to be adulterated with kerosene to reduce its price, it seems.

For some time, Citronella was a popular ingredient in wax candles which helped to deter mosquitos. The oil is used extensively as an ingredient of perfumes, soaps, skin lotions, polishes, detergents and deodorizing cosmetics. Adds an interesting aroma to some Chinese food flavours.

CHEMICAL CONSTITUENTS:
Citronellic (Acid), Borneol, Citronnelol, Geraniol, Nerol (Alcohols), Citral, Citronnelal (Aldehydes), Camphene, Dipentene, Limonene (Terpenes).

PROPERTIES: Antidepressant, Antiseptic, Deodorant, Insecticide, Parasiticide, Tonic, Stimulant.

PRECAUTIONS: ?

MIND: Has a clearing and uplifting effect on the mind which could help ease feelings of depression.

BODY: Its most useful quality appears to be as an insect repellant so perhaps best employed in sprays and diffusers on hot summer days to keep those little pests away. Probably useful in ridding fleas from cats and dogs as well. A drop on cotton wool placed in linen drawers keeps clothes fresh and deters moths and insects.

However it has some reputation for helping to clear the mind and therefore may be effective against headaches, migraine and neuralgia.

It may well act as a general tonic to the body, balancing the heart and nervous system. Could have similar effect on the digestive and reproductive systems, so may be useful at the end of illness to restore tone, spirit and equilibrium. Its antiseptic properties may well be of use in a sick room by keeping germs at bay, again used in a diffuser.

Its deodorant and stimulating qualities could refresh sweaty and tired feet, activating the whole system thereby.

Reputedly helpful for rheumatic aches and pains.

EFFECT ON SKIN: Said to have skin softening qualities when combined with Neroli and Bergamot.

BLENDS: Bergamot, Cajuput, Eucalyptus, Geranium, Lavender, Neroli, Peppermint, Petitgrain, Sage, Ylang Ylang.

CLARY SAGE

Plant/Part	:	Herb/Flowering tops and foliage
Latin Name	:	Salvia sclarea
Family	:	Labiatae
Note	:	Top to Middle
Planet	:	Moon or Mercury
Extraction	:	Distillation

AROMA: A herbal, nutty fragrance, somewhat heavy.

FEATURES: Sclarea is from the Greek 'Skeria' meaning hardness referring to the white/blue flower petals which end in a hard point. A reddish tinged stem, which reaches to about two feet, supports large heart shaped wrinkled leaves. The plant is said to be native to Europe but also found in the United States. Distilled from the fresh herb and oil often comes from France and Morocco.

HISTORY & MYTH: The name also derives from the Latin 'clarus' meaning clear possibly because the herb was once used for clearing mucous from the eyes. Originally grown in southern Europe, it was often planted in German vinyards. When introduced to England in 1562, it was sometimes substituted for hops in brewing beer – with an added intoxicating effect no doubt! In the Middle Ages it was referred to as 'Oculus Christi', meaning eye of Christ. These days often used as an ingredient of perfumes.

CHEMICAL CONSTITUENTS: Linalool, Salviol (Alcohol), Linalyl acetate (Ester), Cineole (Ketone), Caryophyllene (Sesquiterpene).

PROPERTIES: Anticonvulsive, Antidepressant, Antiphlogistic, Antiseptic, Antispasmodic, Antisudorific, Aphrodisiac, Balsamic, Carminative, Deodorant, Digestive, Emmenagogue, Hypotensive, Nervine, Parturient, Sedative, Stomachic, Tonic, Uterine.

PRECAUTIONS: Very sedative and can make concentration difficult – best not to use before driving. Neither should alcohol be taken otherwise a feeling of nausea may result. Large doses can also produce headaches.

MIND: Nervous tension, a racing mind and panicky states could well be eased by this warming and relaxing oil. Its resultant euphoric effect encourages feelings of well being and the capacity to see life in perspective. Excellent pick-me-up for the nerves.

BODY: A good tonic for the womb and particularly helpful with uterine problems. A hormone balancer thereby regulating scanty periods, easing pre menstrual tension and painful cramps in the lower back by helping with muscles to unwind. Seems to have a good reputation with sexual problems by controlling underlying stress and exerts a positive effect on male and female fertility. Also encourages labour, enabling expectant mothers to relax and eases post natal depression.

Soothes digestive problems such as wind and gastric spasm and said to be a good tonic to the kidneys.

May also help headaches and migraine by calming underlying tension. In the same way, its soothing action helps ease the anxiety often associated with muscle spasm and cramp.

Combats excessive perspiration generally and reputedly stems the sweating which accompanies tuberculosis. Said to be useful in treating asthma and sore throats. Strengthens the defence system generally and gives vigour to debilitated states after illness – makes it useful in convalescence.

Its euphoric and uplifting quality may well play a large part in helping people come off drugs by acting as a bridge in those moments of panic and hopelessness. Seems to instill an overall tonic and balancing action on the body.

EFFECT ON SKIN: Appears to possess some cell regenerating properties especially with scalp problems encouraging hair growth. It may clear greasy hair and dandruff by reducing excessive production of sebum. Useful for inflamed and puffy skin.

BLENDS: Bergamot, Cedarwood, Citronella, Cypress, Frankincense, Geranium, Grapefruit, Jasmine, Juniper, Lavender, Lime, Sandalwood.

CLOVE

Plant/Part	:	Tree/Bed
Latin Name	:	Eugenia caryophyllata
Family	:	Myrtaceae
Note	:	Base
Planet	:	Jupiter
Extraction	:	Distillation

AROMA: Strong, spicy and penetrating.

FEATURES: An evergreen columnar shaped tree which grows to about thirty feet. It fares best in clearings rather than in the shade of other trees. The nail shaped flower buds are reddish-brown and the leaves are small and grey. Indigenous to the Molucca Islands and Indonesia, though also cultivated in Zanzibar, Madagascar and Java. Much of the oil is from Sri Lanka.

HISTORY & MYTH: Valued for its medicinal properties by the Greeks, Romans and the Chinese – the latter chewed Cloves to ease toothache and sweeten the breath. The Latin 'Clavus' means nail shaped which the bud resembles. It has a long history as an antiseptic and in prevention of contagious diseases such as the Plague. This was evident when the Dutch destroyed the Clove trees in the Molucca Islands – many epidemics ensued.

It became an important spice imported by the Portuguese and French. Popular use still remains in using oranges studded with Cloves as an aromatic insect repellent. Its aroma makes it a popular ingredient of pot pourri and toothpaste. The digestive properties of this spice are recognised in India though it was also used in love potions. Spicy-toned perfumes often involve Clove and it is also used in mulled wines and liqueurs. The large scale pharmaceutical use recognises its antiseptic and bacteriacidal properties.

CHEMICAL CONSTITUENTS: Furfurol (Aldehyde), Methyl salicylate (Ester), Eugenol (Phenol), Caryophyllene (Sesquiterpene), Pinene (Terpene).

PROPERTIES: Analgesic, Anaesthetic, Antidontalgic, Antiemetic, Antineuralgic, Antiseptic, Antispasmodic, Aperitif, Aphrodisiac, Carminative, Caustic, Cicatrisant, Disinfectant, Insecticide, Parturient, Splenetic, Stimulant, Stomachic, Uterine, Vermifuge.

PRECAUTIONS: A very potent oil and should be used with caution – massage may not be a good medium of application since skin irritation could occur.

MIND: Positive and stimulating effect on the mind, strengthens memory and lifts depression. Uplifting qualities helpful when feeling weak and lethargic.

BODY: Beneficial to the digestive system, renowned for relieving wind by reducing gripping action. Effective against vomiting, diarrhoea, intestinal spasm, dyspepsia, and parasites. Also eases nausea and bad breath due to gastric fermentation. Has a tonic effect on the kidneys, stomach, spleen and intestinal disorders generally.

Its pain relieving properties can help toothache and rheumatism, arthritis and mouth sores as well as tension headaches. Reputedly works best on local areas rather than the system in general.

Relieves respiratory problems and has been used for tuberculosis, asthma and bronchitis. Valuable in disinfecting the atmosphere during infectious illness. An excellent bacteriacide and if frequently vaporised during winter will encourage resistance to germs.

Its aphrodisiac properties may be useful with sexual problems like impotence and frigidity. Consequently giving much pain relief during childbirth apparently.

When mixed with Orange and Lemon, appears to be an excellent insect repellent.

EFFECT ON SKIN: May alleviate infectious wounds, as well as skin sores, leg ulcers and the chronic skin disease lupus.

BLENDS: Basil, Benzoin, Black Pepper, Cinnamon, Citronella, Grapefruit, Lemon, Nutmeg, Orange, Peppermint, Rosemary.

CORIANDER

Plant/Part	:	Herb/Fruit (Seeds)
Latin Name	:	Coriandrum sativum
Family	:	Umbelliferae
Note	:	Top
Planet	:	Venus
Extraction	:	Distillation

AROMA: Slightly pungent, sweet and spicy.

FEATURES: Morocco first gave us this plant though it is now cultivated worldwide, chiefly in the Caucauses, USSR, Armenia and the Mediterranean. The plant's leaves, when crushed, give off an unpleasant odour like squashed bugs, hence the Greek name 'Koris' – for bug and the root wood for Coriander. The brown-grey seeds naturally have a much more pleasant aroma. Grows to about two feet with feathery leaves and pinkish/white flowers.

HISTORY & MYTH: Native of the Middle East and supposedly grown in the Hanging Gardens of Babylon – one of the wonders of the world. Used since ancient times as a medicinal and culinary herb as well as in perfumery. The Egyptians saw it as a spice of happiness probably because it was hailed as an aphrodisiac. The Greeks and Romans flavoured their wines with Coriander as well as using it as a medicinal herb.

In India it was much used in cooking to delay putrefaction of meat though its medicinal value for constipation and insomnia was also recognised as well as an aid in childbearing. Introduced by the Romans into Britain and France. It was an ingredient of a 17th century toilet water produced by the Carmelite Order in Paris, and found its way into liqueurs such as Benedictine and Chartreuse.

CHEMICAL CONSTITUENTS: Borneol, Geraniol, Linalool, Terpineol (Alcohols), Cineole (Ketone), Cymene, Dipentene, Phellandrene, Pinene, Terpinene, Terpinolene (Terpenes).

PROPERTIES: Analgesic, Antispasmodic, Carminative, Deodorant, Depurative, Stimulant, Stomachic.

PRECAUTIONS: Said to be stupefying in large doses.

MIND: A stimulating effect on the mind especially where there is lethargy, fatigue, tension and nervous weakness. Uplifting, refreshing and may help memory and reduce dizziness.

BODY: Mainly acts on the digestive system in relieving wind and stomach cramps. Gives a warming effect on the stomach, stimulates appetite and may help with eating disorders. Seems to have some effect on bad breath.

Since it has a very warming action on the body it can also be used for rheumatic and arthritic pain as well as alleviating muscular spasm. Helpful with cold conditions generally such as influenza and is beneficial to the lungs, reputedly when effected by the measles virus.

Also acts as a general cleanser since it clears the body of toxins and fluid wastes. Its stimulating effect on the body may come through its tonic effect on the spleen, said to be connected to Prana, the life-giving energy. May well be an excellent remedy for exhaustion and feelings of tiredness as well as headaches.

Said to revitalise the glandular system and to stimulate the hormone oestrogen so may redress problems connected to the reproductive system such as irregular periods and infertility.

EFFECT ON SKIN: ?

BLENDS: Bergamot, Black Pepper, Cinnamon, Citronella, Cypress, Galbanum, Geranium, Ginger, Jasmine, Lemon, Melissa, Neroli, Orange.

CUMIN

Plant/Part	:	Herb/Fruit (Seeds)
Latin Name	:	Cuminum cyminum
Family	:	Umbelliferae
Note	:	Top?
Planet	:	Saturn
Extraction	:	Distillation

AROMA: Spicy, penetrating and extremely pungent.

FEATURES: Originally from the Mediterranean region, Egypt and Asia. It reaches to about twelve inches and has deep green, narrow thread-like leaves with tiny white or pink flowers which change to fruit (seed).

HISTORY & MYTH: Held in high esteem since Biblical times, mainly for its digestive properties and used in many meat dishes. The Egyptians included it in a remedy for headaches, along with Juniper and Frankincense and the Pharisees paid tithes (a tax) with it. It was seen as a symbol of fidelity by the Hindus who also valued it as a remedy against jaundice and piles. It was an important ingredient of breadmaking too.

The Greeks and Romans put it in the graves of their dead as well as other gifts. Highly regarded in Britain during the Middle Ages when it was again used as currency – subjects of feudal lords paid with Cumin in lieu of service. Its popularity waned however, upon the introduction of Caraway. It is an essential ingredient in Indian curries and used in Mexico to flavour national dishes. Has some use in perfumery – cannot think why!

CHEMICAL CONSTITUENTS: Cuminic (Aldehyde), Cymene, Dipentene, Limonene, Phellandrene, Pinene (Terpenes).

PROPERTIES: Antiseptic, Antispasmodic, Aphrodisiac, Carminative, Depurative, Digestive, Emmenagogue, Parasiticide, Stimulant, Tonic.

PRECAUTIONS: An overpowering odour, somewhat lingering and best used sparingly. May cause skin sensitisation and should be avoided in pregnancy.

MIND: A strong tonic to the nervous system, it is highly stimulating and acts positively on tiredness and lethargy.

BODY: A very warming oil and relieves toxic congestion in the body. Often found to be helpful with muscular pain and osteoarthritis.

Stimulating effect on the digestion, particularly bloating of the stomach, flatulence, dyspepsia, headaches resulting from stomach disorders, colic and diarrhoea.

Seems to have a beneficial action on the reproductive system since it is said to increase fertility and sexual desire in men. Women benefit too as it appears to normalise the menstrual cycle and increase lactation.

Its tonic action on the heart and nervous system should help regularise the metabolic processes of the body.

EFFECT ON SKIN: ?

BLENDS: Angelica, Caraway, Chamomile, Coriander.

CYPRESS

Plant/Part	:	Tree/Leaves/Cones
Latin Name	:	Cupressus sempervirens
Family	:	Cupresaceae
Note	:	Middle to Base
Planet	:	Saturn
Extraction	:	Distillation

AROMA: Woody and slightly spicy yet clear and refreshing.

FEATURES: The Cypress is a tall, conical shaped tree common to the Mediterranean region. It is a familiar feature in gardens and cemeteries on the Greek islands. An evergreen, it has hard and durable reddish-yellow wood with brown-grey cones. Once cut, apparently, it never grows again though the leaves and branches take longer to die than other species. Oil is often obtained from France and Germany.

HISTORY & MYTH: The Cypress gave its name to the island where it used to be worshipped. It was said that Apollo transformed a young Greek named Cuparissos into the Cypress tree. There is also a legend that the cross was made from the wood and it generally seems to have a connection with death. The Greeks and Romans planted it in their burial grounds and Pluto, god of the underworld, lived in a palace beside which grew the Cypress tree.

It also had many practical uses since the Phoenicians and Cretans used the wood for building houses and ships. The Egyptians employed it for making sarcophagi and various medicinal purposes. The Greeks thought it a good medium for sculpturing statues of their gods possibly because it does not decay easily, hence its name 'Sempervirens' – lives forever. Once an ingredient for whooping cough for children. These days often used in perfumery, particularly for masculine odours.

CHEMICAL CONSTITUENTS: Sabinol (Alcohol), Furfurol (Aldehyde), Terpenyl acetate (Ester), Camphene, Cymene, Pinene, Sylvestrene (Terpenes).

PROPERTIES: Antirheumatic, Antiseptic, Antispasmodic, Antisudorific, Astringent, Cicatrisant, Deodorant, Diuretic, Febrifuge, Haemostatic, Hepatic, Insecticide, Restorative, Sedative, Styptic, Tonic, Vasoconstrictor.

PRECAUTIONS: Regulates the menstrual cycle so best not to use in pregnancy. Its effect on varicose veins is well known, but care should be exercised in applying the oil – actual massage might be too heavy.

MIND: Talkative, irritable people benefit most by its calming action. Seems to have a soothing effect on anger – apparently cleanses the spirit and removes psychic blocks.

BODY: Comes into its own where there is excess of any kind, particularly fluids. Therefore, useful in haemorrhages, oedema, excess bleeding, nose bleeds, heavy menstruation, sweating, particularly of the feet as well as incontinence. May also be beneficial to cellulitis.

With its vaso-constricting effect on the veins, helpful with varicose conditions and haemorrhoids. Acts as a tonic to the circulatory system and also of use where there is excess heat. Its tonic effect on the liver helps to maintain the regular composition of the blood.

Generally has proved helpful with the reproductive system, particularly menstrual problems such pre menstrual tension and the difficult side effects of the menopause, i.e. hot flushes, hormone imbalance and irritability. May regulate ovary dysfunction and has a good effect on painful and heavy periods.

An antispasmodic action can help coughs associated with influenza, bronchitis, whooping cough and asthma. Seems to ease muscular cramps and rheumatism as well.

EFFECT ON SKIN: Exerts a balancing action over fluids. It controls excessive loss of water and can therefore be helpful to the mature skin. Sweaty and oily skin may also benefit and wounds seem to heal well due to its cicatrisant properties.

BLENDS: Benzoin, Bergamot, Clary Sage, Juniper, Lavender, Lemon, Linden Blossom, Orange, Pine, Rosemary, Sandalwood.

DILL

Plant/Part	:	Herb/fruits
Latin Name	:	Anethum graveolens
Family	:	Umbelliferae
Note	:	Top
Planet	:	Mercury
Extraction	:	Distillation

AROMA: Herby, almost grass-like.

FEATURES: A dark green, feathery leaved plant said to originate from India. With its small yellow flowers and tiny compressed fruits, it looks a bit like Fennel but does not grow as tall. These days it is found in the Mediterranean region, Europe and the Black Sea. The Indian oil differs from the European variety in its chemical composition.

HISTORY & MYTH: Apparently first heard of in Egypt about 5,000 years ago where it was mixed with Coriander and Bryony to ease headaches. It was popular with the Greeks and Romans who called it 'Anethon', from which the botanical name is derived. Believed by some that it is the 'Anise' mentioned in the Bible (Matthew 23,23), since it was widely cultivated in Palestine. Ancient medics believed it was good for hiccups.

The name Dill evolved from the Anglo-Saxon Dylle or Dylla, which had changed by the medieval period to Dill – meaning lull, probably referring to its principal use as a carminative though also used in compresses for insomnia. There is an old icelandic word Dilla which refers to soothing a child. Became a very common plant in the Middle Ages, believed to be a charm against witchcraft and was popular in love potions. In 812 Charlemagne, Emperor of France, ordered extensive cultivation of the plant. Often used in fish dishes, breads, soups, sauces and pickling gherkins.

CHEMICAL CONSTITUENTS: Carvone (Ketone), Eugenol, Myristicin (Phenols), Limonene, Phellandrene, Terpinene (Terpenes).

PROPERTIES: Antispasmodic, Carminative, Digestive, Disinfectant, Galactogogue, Parturient, Sedative, Stomachic, Sudorific.

PRECAUTIONS: Once used to ease childbirth so perhaps best avoided during pregnancy.

MIND: Helpful when feeling overwhelmed and may be of use in shock and times of crises. Gives one space to be, as well as inducing a lightness of feeling and allowing cares to fall away.

BODY: Dillwater (Gripe) often helps children's digestive disorders, particularly wind in the stomach or bowels. The oil is much more powerful however, and should not be used on infants.

Yet could be helpful for disordered digestion in adults, easing flatulence and constipation. May have an effect on gastric fermentation and gets rid of bad breath. Seems to ease hiccups probably due to its antispasmodic properties.

Said to promote flow of mother's milk and its efficacy in easing childbirth may still prevail.

Seems to calm nervous states which are accompanied by throbbing headaches and excess sweating.

EFFECT ON SKIN: Promotes healing of wounds.

BLENDS: Bergamot, Coriander, Cypress, Geranium, Mandarin, Myrtle, Orange, Petitgrain, Rosemary.

ELEMI

Plant/Part	:	Tree/Bark
Latin Name	:	Canarium luzonicum
Family	:	Burseraceae
Note	:	Base
Planet	:	Sun?
Extraction	:	Distillation

AROMA: Citrus-like and a little spicy.

FEATURES: A tree from the Philippines which exudes a natural resin subsequently yielding a rather exotic essential oil. It is only when the tree sprouts leaves that the pale yellow resin is produced – it solidifies on contact with the air – and stops when the last leaf falls. It was known locally as 'Pili' though sometimes referred to as 'Manila Elemi'. However, there are other varieties of Elemi, i.e. 'Protum Heptaphyllum' from Brazil, 'Amyris Plumerrii' from Mexico etc.

HISTORY & MYTH: Popular in Europe since 15th century, often used in old fashioned unguents, though still employed in medicinal preparations and pharmaceutical plasters. An ingredient of incense, soaps and apparently capable of applying a toughness to varnishes. The crude gum is exported from Manila in two qualities: 'Primera' which is cleaned gum or 'Secunda' crude, uncleaned gum. Chemical examination of the oil began late last century.

CHEMICAL CONSTITUENTS: Terpineol (Alcohol), Elemicine (Phenol), Elemol (Sesquiterpene), Dipentene, Limonene, Phellandrene (Terpenes).

PROPERTIES: Analgesic, Antiviral, Bacteriacide, Balsamic, Expectorant, Fungicide, Tonic, Vulnerary.

PRECAUTIONS: Possibly irritant to sensitive skins.

MIND: Seems to have a grounding yet joyous effect, instills a feeling of peace and may well be a helpful nerve sedative.

BODY: Appears to have a strengthening effect on the body through its immuno stimulant properties. Possibly helpful at the start of illness in order to fortify the body in fighting disease.

Catarrhal conditions respond well and Elemi seems to have a regulating energy on cold conditions generally. May well ease congestion of the lungs and control excess mucous.

Apparently helps to stem overflow of bodily secretions such as perspiration.

It is also credited in having a tonic and clearing effect on the urinary system.

EFFECT ON SKIN: Said to be similar to Myrrh, that is cooling and drying on the skin. Also reputedly helpful for chronic skin conditions such as ulcers, fungal growths and infected wounds. Could well have a balancing effect on sebum.

BLENDS: Cardamom, Frankincense, Galbanum, Geranium, Ginger, Lavender, Litsea Cubeba, Melissa, Orange, Rosewood.

EUCALYPTUS

Plant/Part	:	Tree/Leaves
Latin Name	:	Eucalyptus globulus
Family	:	Myrtaceae
Note	:	Top
Planet	:	?
Extraction	:	Distillation

AROMA: Clear, sharp and piercing.

FEATURES: Eucalyptus, the Australian gum-tree, reaches an imposing height. It is something like three-hundred feet with tough scimitar-shaped leaves. A tendency to grow in malarial countries helps to drain the land producing a healthier climate. The oil is distilled from several varieties of Eucalyptus tree which dominate the Australian flora. Other varieties are E. Polybractrea, E. Dumosa and E. Radiata, the latter having more cooling properties apparently and a more camphor-like aroma. E. Maculata and E. Citriodora incline to a citrus-like aroma.

HISTORY & MYTH: The 'eu' and 'kalypto' is of Greek origin, meaning 'well' and 'cover' referring to the covered stamens. The Australian Aborigines called it 'Kino' and bound the leaves around serious wounds. It was introduced into Europe as an ornamental species around 1788 and was found to inhibit the growth of other plants in surrounding areas due to secreting a chemical poison into the soil. The first Eucalyptus oil exported to England – from Eucalyptus piperita – was known as 'Sydney Peppermint' due to its soothing action on digestive complaints.

CHEMICAL CONSTITUENTS: Citronellal (Aldehyde), Cineole (Ketone), Camphene, Fenchene, Phellandrene, Pinene (Terpenes).

PROPERTIES: Analgesic, Antirheumatic, Antiphlogistic, Antiseptic, Antispasmodic, Antiviral, Bactericide, Balsamic, Cicatrisant, Decongestant, Deodorant, Depurative, Diuretic, Expectorant, Febrifuge, Hypoglycemiant, Insecticide, Rubefacient, Stimulant, Vermifuge, Vulnerary.

PRECAUTIONS: A powerful oil so care should be taken with dosage. Best avoided on people suffering from high blood pressure or epilepsy. May antidote homeopathic medication.

MIND: Has a cooling effect upon the emotions. Also clears the head, aids concentration and strengthens the nervous system.

BODY: Its anti-viral action works well on the respiratory tract, soothing inflammation and easing mucous. Particularly good for influenza, throat infections, coughs, catarrhal conditions, sinusitis, asthma and tuberculosis. Clears the head due to stuffiness from colds and hay fever. Excellent with infectious illnesses.

Effective in all types of fever, lowers the temperature, has a cooling and deodorising action upon the body. May reduce painful effects of migraine and reputedly helpful with scarlet fever, dysentery, typhoid, diphtheria and malaria as well as chicken pox.

Works well on the genito-urinary system dealing with such problems as cystitis as well as diarrhoea. Seems to dissolve gall stones and has been used to treat nephritis, gonorrhoea and diabetes. Said to be effective against haemorrhage.

Some relief may be obtained from rheumatism – said to be effective when combined with Lemon and Juniper. May also be helpful with general muscular aches and pains, and neuralgia (nerve pain) as well as pyorrhoea.

Said to antidote bites from insects as well as other venomous creatures.

EFFECTS ON SKIN: Apparently useful for skin eruptions like herpes and good for burns, preventing bacterial growth and subsequent pus formation aiding construction of new tissue. Cuts, wounds, ulcers and inflammatory conditions also seem to respond well. Clears congested skin.

BLENDS: Benzoin, Coriander, Juniper, Lavender, Lemon, Lemongrass, Melissa, Pine, Thyme.

FENNEL

Plant/Part	:	Herb/Seeds
Latin Name	:	Foeniculum vulgare
Family	:	Umbelliferae
Note	:	Top to middle
Planet	:	Mercury
Extraction	:	Distillation

AROMA: Floral, herby and slightly spicy.

FEATURES: Not to be confused with Florence Fennel which is a vegetable. Our F. vulgare, with its yellow flowers is very attractive to bees. It also has bushy green feathery leaves, oblong fruits and reaches to about five feet. Found growing in the Mediterranean where much of the oil comes from. 'Foeniculum' is from the Latin 'Foenum' meaning 'hay'.

HISTORY & MYTH: A very popular plant with the ancient Chinese who used it as a cure for snake bite. The Egyptians and Romans recognised its stomachic and anti-toxic properties and saw it as an emblem of flattery as well. The herb was also thought to be helpful for various afflictions to the eyes, especially cataracts. It did a neat trick in expelling worms from ears too.

It was also popular as a slimming aid since it gave a feeling of fullness. Like Dill, it was used in 'Gripewater' to help infants' colic. In mediaeval times it was known as 'Fenkle' and was thought to ward off evil spirits and dog fleas. Since it was often planted near kennels we can presume that dogs remained free of fleas and suitably exorcised!

CHEMICAL CONSTITUENTS: Anisic, Cuminic (Aldehydes), Fenchone (Ketone), Anethole, Methylchavicol (Phenols), Camphene, Dipentene, Limonene, Phellandrene (Terpenes).

PROPERTIES: Antiphlogistic, Antiseptic, Antispasmodic, Aperitif, Carminative, Detoxicant, Diuretic, Emmenagogue, Expectorant, Galactagogue, Insecticide, Laxative, Resolvent, Splenetic, Stimulant, Stomachic, Sudorific, Tonic, Vermifuge.

PRECAUTIONS: A powerful oil, easily subject to toxicity with over-use. May cause skin sensitisation. Best avoided in pregnancy and people suffering from epilepsy should stay clear of it.

MIND: An oil said to give strength and courage in adversity. Some say it bestows longevity.

BODY: An excellent body cleanser, ridding the system of poisonous toxins resulting from excess food and alcohol. It is great for hangovers acting as a tonic to the liver, kidneys and spleen. Clears poisons from insect and serpent bites too! Helpful in reducing diets as it seems effective in dispersing cellulitis through its diuretic action. May also dissolve kidney stones.

Works well on stomach ailments since it is a tonic to the digestion. It eases indigestion when eating under stress by calming the nervous system. Good for hiccups, nausea, vomiting and colic. A clearing action on the intestines helps to relieve constipation and flatulence.

As an antispasmodic and expectorant, may be useful in cold conditions and bronchitis as well as whooping cough.

Said to activate the glandular system by imitating the hormone oestrogen. This could make it helpful with pre menstrual tension, scanty periods, menopausal problems and low sexual response. Well known for increasing milk in nursing mothers.

EFFECT ON SKIN: Seems to have a cleansing and tonic action on the skin and a reputation for keeping wrinkles at bay!

BLENDS: Basil, Geranium, Lavender, Lemon, Rose, Rosemary, Sandalwood.

FIR

Plant/Part	:	Tree/Needles/Leaves
Latin Name	:	Abies balsamea Abies sibirica
Family	:	Pinaceae
Note	:	Middle
Planet	:	Jupiter
Extraction	:	Distillation

AROMA: Clear, balsamic and refreshing.

FEATURES: The many species of Fir, growing mainly in northern climes, usually have leathery, herring-bone branches bearing cones. Some species are also found as far south as Mexico and Algeria. The resin type oil generally obtained from A. balsamea, comes from America and Canada. A. sibirica – known as Siberian Fir – is grown in Russia the older needles producing the most oil. Another species, the Grand Fir (Abies Grandis) emits a strong smell of oranges when bruised.

HISTORY & MYTH: Early this century many small village industries still produced this oil on a rather large scale in Russia. The biblical 'Balm of Gilead' is A. Balsamea, and was a tree often employed in house and shipbuilding due to its durability. The native American Indians used the resin for medicinal and religious purposes and it was introduced into Europe some time during 17th century. Its many uses include toilet and shaving soaps bath preparations, room sprays, deodorants, disinfectants and inhalations.

CHEMICAL CONSTITUENTS: Bornyl acetate, Terpinyl acetate (Esters), Bisabolene, Camphene, Dipentene, Phellandrene, Pinene (Terpenes).

PROPERTIES: Antiscorbutic, Antiseptic, Expectorant, Pectoral, Sedative.

PRECAUTIONS: So far not used overmuch in Aromatherapy, perhaps because the contraindications are uncertain.

MIND: May have a warming and grounding effect.

BODY: Its most helpful action seems to be on the respiratory system and appears to have a beneficial effect on chest conditions especially obstructions of the bronchi such as fluid, pus and mucous. Deals very well with shortness of breath and could be of use to asthma sufferers, particularly since it has a tonic effect on the nervous system as well. Relieves tiredness and aching limbs which often accompany colds and influenza.

Its warming action may be a palliative for muscular aches and pains due to rheumatic or arthritic conditions.

Acts as a urinary antiseptic and could be helpful with infections.

Also appears to invigorate the endocrine glands which could favourably affect the metabolic rate balancing the chemical reactions in the body.

EFFECT ON SKIN: ?

BLENDS: Basil, Caraway, Cedarwood, Frankincense, Lavender, Myrtle, Niaouli, Rosewood.

FRANKINCENSE

Plant/Part	:	Tree/Bark
Latin Name	:	Boswellia carteri/thurifera
Family	:	Burseraceae
Note	:	Middle to Base
Planet	:	Sun
Extraction	:	Distillation

AROMA: A haunting fragrance, woody, spicy with a hint of lemon.

FEATURES: The tree originates from the Middle East, mainly China, Ethiopia, Iran and the Lebanon. Incisions are made in the tree bark which exudes resin in yellow drops or tears from which the oil is distilled.

HISTORY & MYTH: 'Frank' in French means 'real incense' though sometimes referred to as Olibanum, probably signifying Oil from Lebanon. It was burnt at altars in Egypt as an offering to the gods and used as an aid to meditation, a tradition still in practise in some religions. At one stage, it was also used to fumigate the sick in an effort to banish evil spirits.

The Egyptians would often incorporate it with Cinnamon to soothe aching limbs. Indeed the Hebrews and Egyptians spent a fortune importing it from the Phoenicians. Such was its value in those days – almost as much as gold – that it was offered as a gift to the infant Jesus. The Egyptians employed it cosmetically in rejuvenating masks and the Chinese found it helpful in treating scrofula – tuberculosis of the lymph glands – as well as leprosy. These days it is used as a fixative in perfumes.

CHEMICAL CONSTITUENTS: Cadinene (Sesquiterpene), Camphene, Dipentene, Pinene, Phellandrene (Terpenes), Olibanol (Alcohol).

PROPERTIES: Antiseptic, Astringent, Carminative, Cicatrisant, Cytophylactic, Digestive, Diuretic, Sedative, Tonic, Uterine, Vulnerary.

PRECAUTIONS: ?

MIND: Slows down breathing producing feelings of calm. This tends to bring about an elevating and soothing effect on the mind. Its comforting and somewhat refreshing action is helpful for anxious and obsessional states linked to the past.

BODY: Has a pronounced effect on the mucous membranes, particularly helpful in clearing the lungs. Excellent effect on respiration, eases shortness of breath and useful to asthma sufferers. Good remedy for catarrhal conditions and generally regulates secretions. Has a soothing action on head colds and a palliative for coughs, bronchitis and laryngitis.

Seems to have a helpful action on the genito-urinary tract and may mitigate the effects of cystitis, nephritis and genital infections generally.

Its astringent properties may relieve uterine haemorrhages as well as heavy periods and generally acts as a tonic to the uterus. Said to be of value during labour with its calming action and could ease post natal depression. May also treat breast inflammation.

Also soothes the stomach, easing digestion, dyspepsia and belching!

EFFECT ON SKIN: Gives new life to ageing skin and reputedly smooths out wrinkles! A real tonic to the skin. Its astringent properties may also help balance oily conditions. Found to be effective with wounds, sores, ulcers, carbuncles and inflammation.

BLENDS: Basil, Black Pepper, Galbanum, Geranium, Grapefruit, Lavender, Orange, Melissa, Patchouli, Pine, Sandalwood.

GALBANUM

Plant/Part	:	Shrub/Bark
Latin Name	:	Ferula galbaniflua
Family	:	Umbelliferae
Note	:	Top
Planet	:	Sun
Extraction	:	Distillation

AROMA: Musk-like, evocative of damp woodlands and fresh poppy seeds.

FEATURES: A shrub found in the Middle East, particularly Iran and Levant producing hard and soft resin respectively. The oil is distilled from this pale green gum which exudes naturally from the tree or from cuts made from the base of shoots. The Iranian oil seems to have a more Turpentine-like odour. Another species, F. ceratophylla, from Turkestan produces an oil from the flowers.

HISTORY & MYTH: A celebrated incense of ancient times which indicates a rather mystical influence. It has a slightly narcotic effect and often used as an aid to meditation. Certainly it was a popular ingredient in holy oil. The Bible speaks of it being employed as such in Exodus 30:34 where it is combined with Frankincense as well as Onycha and Stacte for use in the Tabernacle.

The Egyptians used it as an ingredient for embalming indicating its strong preservative properties. These days employed as a fixative and an ingredient for oriental type perfumes. Dr Arnould Taylor in 'Aromatherapy for the Whole Person' mentions that it is an oil preferably to be used on the elderly rather than the young.

CONSTITUENTS: Borneol, Guaiol, Linalool, Terpineol (Alcohols), Carvone (Ketone), Cadinene, Cadinol (Sesquiterpenes), Carene, Limonene, Myrcene, Pinene, Terpinolene (Terpenes).

PROPERTIES: Analgesic, Antispasmodic, Carminative, Diuretic, Emmenagogue, Expectorant, Resolvent, Vulnerary, Stimulant.

PRECAUTIONS: An emmenagogue so best avoided in pregnancy. The lingering aroma can be a bit 'heady' and could induce headaches as well as irritate mucous membranes. Possibility of some skin irritation too.

MIND: May well have a grounding effect due to its reputation in removing psychic blockages. Seems to calm erratic moods and ease nervous tension.

BODY: Usually effective on hard to shift ailments and could be a force against chronic conditions generally.

It has long been used for persistent infection of the lungs especially good for freeing mucous and easing troublesome coughs. On the whole beneficial to the respiratory tract especially in calming bronchial spasm.

A boon to the reproductive system dealing with problems such as lack of periods, menstrual cramp and water retention. Menopausal difficulties involving irritable moods and hot flushes could be made more bearable.

Its analgesic and antispasmodic action may help with muscle cramp and rheumatism.

EFFECT ON SKIN: Beneficial in cases of inflammation, swellings, wounds and abscesses particularly those conditions which respond to little else. May also help to soften mature skins.

BLENDS: Citronella, Elemi, Frankincense, Jasmine, Palmarosa, Geranium, Ginger, Pine, Rose, Tagetes, Verbena, Ylang Ylang.

GARLIC

Plant/Part	:	Herb/Stem and pods
Latin Name	:	Allium sativum
Family	:	Liliaceae
Note	:	?
Planet	:	Mars
Extraction	:	Distillation

AROMA: Strong acrid odour.

FEATURES: The Celtic 'Allium' refers to the plant's powerful 'burning' essence. Originally from Asia but also grows in Spain, Egypt, Sicily and France. It reaches to about three feet and has white or pink flowers with long flat leaves. The white bulb is composed of cloves with membranous tracts.

HISTORY & MYTH: Has a reputation for bestowing longevity. Phoenician sailors carried huge stocks of garlic on long sea voyages to avert disease. The Egyptians employed it against epidemics like cholera and typhus and the ancient Greeks thought it effective against sterility. Greek wrestlers would chew a few cloves of garlic before fighting bouts to give themselves strength and courage and no doubt to deter their opponents. Also used extensively in Chinese medicine.

Its reputation in guarding against witchcraft is upheld by Vampires who we all know are not too fond of it. Indeed the Swedes also believed it kept the 'trolls' – mischievous nordic goblins – in their place. French country folk used Garlic to ward off predators. Both World Wars saw the widespread use of Garlic for its antibiotic properties.

CHEMICAL CONSTITUENTS: Diallyl disulphide, Allyl disulfide (Sulphur Compounds).

PROPERTIES: Analgesic, Antibiotic, Antisclerotic, Antiparasitic, Antiseptic, Antispasmodic, Antiviral, Bacteriacide, Cholagogue, Cicatrisant, Decongestant, Diuretic, Escharotic, Expectorant, Fungicide, Hypoglycemiant, Hypotensive, Insecticide, Prophylactic, Resolvent, Sudorific, Tonic, Vasodilator, Vermifuge.

PRECAUTIONS: Garlic is 'fiery' in nature and best avoided by people who are either angry or heated. Neither should it be used on acute pulmonary and digestive conditions – its rapid detoxifying nature may be a bit of a shock to the body. Also indicated against skin disorders like eczema which could point to a metabolic disorder. Babies could get colic if used by nursing mothers. Most people prefer to take garlic capsules rather than use it in Aromatherapy massage.

MIND: Its warming and stimulating properties dispel tiredness.

BODY: A tonic to the body and strengthens the constitution. Retards the ageing process mainly by its regulating effect on the thyroid gland which influences cell production. Tones up the lymphatic system encouraging detoxification.

Very helpful to the circulatory system. By dilating the capillaries it brings down blood pressure and reduces high cholesterol levels by its action on the metabolism of fats and has a tonic and balancing effect on circulation. Helps to thin the blood and can control hardening of the arteries.

An affinity with the respiratory tract makes it effective against influenza, laryngitis, chest complaints and bronchial catarrh. Has been used to relieve tuberculosis, diphtheria, chronic bronchitis and whooping cough.

Beneficial to the digestive tract by stimulating peristalsis and working as a laxative. Also checks fermentation and putrefaction in the stomach and casts out worms. Stimulates the gall bladder to promote bile flow, helping digestion of fats. Seems to have an effect on insulin regulation and might be valuable in diabetes. Its diuretic action guards against kidney stones.

Soothes sprains, muscular and rheumatic pains as well as neuritis.

EFFECT ON SKIN: Indicated for various skin problems such as spots, acne, abscess, ringworm and lupus. Used for disinfecting ulcers and septic wounds. Corns and warts may respond.

BLENDS: ?

GERANIUM

Plant/Part	:	Flowering plant/ Flowers and leaves
Latin Name	:	Pelargonium odorantissimum/ graveolens
Family	:	Geraniaceae
Note	:	Middle
Planet	:	Venus
Extraction	:	Distillation

AROMA: Sweet and heavy, a little like rose with minty overtones.

FEATURES: This attractive plant, often seen in hedgerows, is about two feet high with serrated, pointed leaves and small pink flowers. The oil is often obtained from France, Reunion, Spain, Morocco, Egypt and Italy. Geranium is a misnomer since the oil is really derived from Pelargoniums. P. Odorantissimum may have a slight apple-like fragrance where P. Graveolens favours a rose aroma.

HISTORY & MYTH: Once regarded as a great healing plant and often used as a remedy for wounds, tumours, cholera and fractures. Indeed, belief in its powers throughout the centuries disposed people to plant it around their cottages to keep evil spirits at bay!

The French began commercial production of Geranium oil early in 19th century though much of the oil today comes from Reunion, formerly called Bourbon, an aromatic island in the South western Indian Ocean. The first species used was probably P. capitatum, a smaller plant apparently yielding a high percentage of oil and still continues to grow wild. Early this century Morocco began to compete in production of Geranium oil. A fragrance often used in perfumes and soaps and can be made to imitate most fragrances.

CHEMICAL CONSTITUENTS: Geranic (Acid), Geraniol, Citronellol, Linalool, Myrtenol, Terpineol (Alcohols), Citral (Aldehyde), Methone (Ketone), Eugenol (Phenol), Sabinene (Terpene).

PROPERTIES: Analgesic, Anticoagulant, Antidepressant, Antiseptic, Astringent, Cicatrisant, Cytophylactic, Diuretic, Deodorant, Haemostatic, Hypoglycemiant, Insecticide, Styptic, Tonic, Vasoconstrictor, Vulnerary.

PRECAUTIONS: May cause some irritation to sensitive skins. Regulates the hormonal system so may not be a good idea to use in pregnancy.

MIND: A tonic to the nervous system, quells anxiety and depression and lifts the spirits. Puts the mind back into balance and through its action on the adrenal cortex reduces stress.

BODY: With its regulatory function on the hormonal system, useful with pre menstrual tension and menopausal problems such as depression, lack of vaginal secretion and heavy periods. Said to be helpful with inflammation and congestion of the breasts.

Its diuretic properties are very effective when general elimination is poor and the system congested. A tonic action on the liver and kidneys helps to clear the body of toxins which may be a source of help for addictions. Also deals with such problems as jaundice, kidney and gall bladder stones, diabetes and urinary infections. Generally helps guard against fluid retention and swollen ankles.

Also has a stimulating effect on the lymphatic system which keeps infection at bay and disposes of waste products. It is also a tonic to the circulation, making it more fluid.

Effective in throat and mouth infections – if the sweet aromatic flavour appeals. Its pain relieving qualities also helps ease neuralgia.

Generally has a clearing effect on mucous, mainly of the digestive system and may be good for gastritis and colitis.

An aromatic insect repellent.

EFFECT ON SKIN: Useful for all types of skin conditions since it balances sebum, the fatty secretion in sebaceous glands which keeps the skin supple. Eczema, burns, shingles, herpes, ringworm and chilblains may respond. Also good for sluggish, congested and oily skins – a good overall skin cleanser. Livens up pale skins since Geranium improves the flow of blood.

BLENDS: Angelica, Basil, Bay, Bergamot, Carrot Seed, Cedarwood, Citronella, Clary Sage, Grapefruit, Jasmine, Lavender, Lime, Neroli, Orange, Petitgrain, Rose, Rosemary, Sandalwood.

GINGER

Plant/Part	:	Herb/Rhizome
Latin Name	:	Zingiber officinale
Family	:	Zingiberaceae
Note	:	Top
Planet	:	Mars
Extraction	:	Distillation

AROMA: Spicy, sharp, warm and pleasant, very alive with a hint of lemon and pepper.

FEATURES: Grown commercially in most tropical countries like Africa and the West Indies, though said to be native to India, China and Java. Jamaica Ginger boasts the best aroma apparently. It is a perennial herb, has an erect reed-like white flowering stem rising from a creeping jointed root.

HISTORY & MYTH: A spice highly esteemed throughout the ages and included in the ancient Greek and Arab pharmacopoeia. The dried root was a popular condiment, aromatic stimulant and a remedy against malaria. The Chinese used it to break up phlegm and strengthen the heart.

There is some uncertainty about its introduction to Europe, possibly the 10th or 15th century, but there is no mystery about its identity – it seems to have been baptised several times. The Greeks called it 'Ziggiber' and favoured its warming properties on the stomach and as an antidote to poison. It was listed in Sanskrit writings as 'Srngavera' and also reputedly named Ginger from the Latin Zingiber. Last but not least, it is also said that the name derives from the Gingi district in India, where the tea is taken for stomach upsets.

CHEMICAL CONSTITUENTS: Borneol (Alcohol), Citral (Aldehyde), Cineole (Ketone), Zingiberene (Sesquiterpene), Camphene, Limonene, Phellandrene (Terpenes).

PROPERTIES: Analgesic, Antiemetic, Antiseptic, Antiscorbutic, Aperitif, Aphrodisiac, Carminative, Expectorant, Febrifuge, Laxative, Rubefacient, Stimulant, Stomachic, Sudorific, Tonic.

PRECAUTIONS: Could irritate sensitive skins.

MIND: Warming to the emotions when feeling flat and cold. It sharpens the senses and aids memory. Very cheering and indicated for tiredness. Stimulating yet grounding too.

BODY: Especially helpful where there is excess of moisture as in catarrh, influenza and runny colds. Sore throats and tonsillitis can also be eased. Though a warming oil tending to counteract ailments caused by dampness, is also able to reduce feverish conditions by increasing activity of sweat glands subsequently cooling the body down. Reputedly helpful in regulating menstruation when effected by colds.

Tones and settles the digestive system promoting secretion of gastric juices. Loss of appetite, painful digestion, flatulence, diarrhoea and scurvy (an incorrect diet lacking in vitamin C) seem to respond favourably to this oil. Also effective against feelings of nausea, hangovers, travel and sea sickness.

Its analgesic properties relieve arthritic and rheumatic pains as well as cramp, sprains and muscle spasm especially in the lower back.

Stimulates the circulation and may ease angina – a painful strangling sensation in the heart region. Said to help reduce chilblains, high cholesterol levels in the blood and varicose veins.

Long hailed as an aphrodisiac and seemingly a valuable remedy in cases of impotence – a blend with Cinnamon, Coriander and Rosemary works wonders apparently. As a possible consequence of this it is said to be helpful after childbirth, breaking down remaining clots.

Reputedly good for the eyesight – though no essential oil of course should be used directly on this delicate area. Said to improve hearing and generally sharpens the senses.

EFFECT ON SKIN: Helpful in clearing bruising, sores and carbuncles.

BLENDS: Bay, Cajuput, Caraway, Cardamom, Cinnamon, Coriander, Clove, Elemi, Eucalyptus, Frankincense, Geranium, Lemon, Lime, Myrtle, Orange, Rosemary, Spearmint, Verbena.

GRAPEFRUIT

Plant/Part	:	Tree/Peel
Latin Name	:	Citrus paradisi
Family	:	Rutaceae
Note	:	Top
Planet	:	?
Extraction	:	Expression

AROMA: Sweet, sharp and refreshing.

FEATURES: A glossy leaved tree with white flowers and yellow fruits which hang from the trees like large bunches of grapes flattened at the ends. The oil glands are embedded deep within the peel and compared to Orange and Lemon, the yield of oil is small. Some Grapefruit oil is obtained by distillation but the quality is apparently inferior compared to the expressed variety. Much of the essential oil is obtained from Israel, Brazil and the USA.

HISTORY & MYTH: Often grown in the Mediterranean as an ornamental tree though its origins from Asia however, are said to result from a hybrid of Orange. Other rumours assert that the fruit was first cultivated in the West Indies some time during the 18th century. It was then known as 'shaddock fruit', so named apparently after the Captain who introduced the fruit to that part of the world. Primary commercialism of essential oil was in Florida about 1930 and it is the USA which remains the largest supplier. A popular ingredient in food, cosmetics and perfumes.

CHEMICAL CONSTITUENTS: Geraniol, Linalool (Alcohol), Citral (Aldehyde), Limonene, Pinene (Terpenes).

PROPERTIES: Antidepressant, Antiseptic, Aperitif, Diuretic, Disinfectant, Resolvent, Stimulant, Tonic.

PRECAUTIONS: Skin irritation could occur if exposed to strong sunlight after treatment.

MIND: Has an overall uplifting and reviving effect making it valuable in states of stress. May well have a balancing action on the central nervous system since bears a reputation for stabilizing manic-depression. Said to be euphoric and slightly hypnotic.

BODY: A lymphatic stimulant, nourishes the tissue cells and controls liquid processes. It may have an effect on obesity and water retention and its diuretic properties could help with cellulite. As an aid to weight reducing diets, it stimulates bile secretion helping with digestion of fats.

However, it is an appetite stimulant too indicating its general balancing and tonic effect on the digestion. Could be an aid in drug withdrawal since it is said to have a cleansing effect on the kidneys and vascular system. Its dissolving quality could diffuse gall stones. Said to be a tonic to the liver too.

Appears to have a soothing effect on the body since it is said to relieve migraine, pre menstrual tension and uncomfortable feelings during pregnancy. It also seems to mitigate some of the effects of jet lag i.e. headaches and tiredness.

May help to restore balance after ear infections.

EFFECT ON SKIN: ?

BLENDS: Basil, Bergamot, Cedarwood, Chamomile, Citronella, Frankincense, Geranium, Jasmine, Lavender, Palmarosa, Rose, Rosewood, Ylang Ylang.

GUAIACWOOD

Plant/Part	:	Tree/Heartwood
Latin Name	:	Guaiacum officinale, G. sanctum Bulnesia sarmienti
Family	:	Zygophyllaceae
Note	:	Base
Planet	:	?
Extraction	:	Distillation

AROMA: Deep, strong and earthy with smoky vanilla undertones.

FEATURES: Originally from South America, B. sarmienta seems to yield the greatest quantity of the oil-resin. Though some oil is obtained from G. sanctum which comes from South Florida and The Bahamas. A small tree, about twelve feet with light green leaves, white bark, greeny-brown heartwood and blue flowers. The wood is usually sold in shavings or raspings. Although the resin exudes quite naturally, it is sometimes produced by firing the logs and collecting the melted resin. The oil is solid at room temperature and may need to be heated before it will melt.

HISTORY & MYTH: Sometimes known as 'Paolo Santo' or 'Holy Tree' indicating possible use in magical/religious ceremonies. The people of Paraguay however, saw its worth in the treatment of serious diseases such as cancer and syphilis – probably due to its 'sweating' properties.

The hardwood is used for carving bowls and other decorative ornaments. First shipped to Europe for extraction of oil around 1891, though distillation in Paraguay began just before the outbreak of the Second World War. Its fixative value is recognised in perfumes and many years ago it was used as an adulterant for Rose Otto. An ingredient of soap when rose compositions are used.

CHEMICAL CONSTITUENTS: Bulnesol, Guaiol (Alcohols).

PROPERTIES: Antiphlogistic, Antirheumatic, Aphrodisiac, Astringent, Balsamic, Diuretic, Laxative, Sudorific.

PRECAUTIONS: May produce a languid feeling impeding concentration and the aroma tends to linger which may not appeal to everyone.

MIND: A relaxing, surrendering quality helpful for meditation. Possibly relieves nervous tension.

BODY: Its first-rate sudorific properties help expel impurities of the blood. Has a long standing use for gout and rheumatoid arthritis – particularly helpful where there is inflammation. By the same token, it promotes perspiration with feverish colds, is soothing to the mucous membranes of the throat and may ease tonsillitis.

Could generally have a tonic effect on the bodily fluids, may be helpful with sexual difficulties, i.e. lack of vaginal secretions during menopause which lead to painful intercourse. Its earthy and mysterious quality could mean it lives up to its reputation as an aphrodisiac! It may also soothe painful periods.

A positive effect on a sluggish genito-urinary system gets things moving again acting as a diuretic and laxative.

EFFECT ON SKIN: Seems to tighten tissues and may be of assistance to mature skins.

BLENDS: Benzoin, Bergamot, Celery, Citronella, Elemi, Frankincense, Geranium, Grapefruit, Jasmine, Lavender, Lemon, Palmarosa, Patchouli, Rose, Ylang Ylang.

HYSSOP

Plant/Part	:	Herb/Leaves and Flowering tops
Latin Name	:	Hyssopus officinalis
Family	:	Labiatae
Note	:	Middle
Planet	:	Jupiter
Extraction	:	Distillation

AROMA: Warm, sweet and penetrating.

FEATURES: The purple/blue flowers, which decorate the Mediterranean flora, are very attractive to bees. Hyssop grows to about two feet high and has hairy, woody stems with slender green leaves. Oil often obtained from Germany, France and Italy.

HISTORY & MYTH: The quote from the Bible: 'Purge me with Hyssop and I shall be clean', Psalm 51:7 may well refer to the plant's general cleansing effect in connection with plagues, leprosy and chest ailments. Indeed, its deodorant properties were employed in cleansing and refreshing holy temples and was long held to be a sacred plant. It was on a twig of Hyssop that a sponge filled with vinegar was handed to Jesus on the cross – John 19:20. The name is derived from the Hebrew 'Ezoph' and Green 'Azob'.

Probably introduced into Europe about 10th century by Benedictine monks who used it as an ingredient of liqueurs. It was one of the strewing herbs of the middle ages which was used to ward off lice. The leaves were sometimes bound over wounds and apparently brought rapid healing. Pulverised powder made from Hyssop helped swellings and spots and was also used to treat cancerous growths.

CHEMICAL CONSTITUENTS: Borneol, Linalool (Alcohols), Camphor, Pinocamphone, Thujone (Ketones), Cadinene (Sesquiterpene), Camphene, Pinene (Terpenes).

PROPERTIES: Antirheumatic, Antiseptic, Antispasmodic, Astringent, Bechic, Cardiac, Carminative, Cephalic, Cicatrisant, Digestive, Diuretic, Emmenagogue, Expectorant, Febrifuge, Emollient, Hypertensive, Nervine, Pectoral, Prophylactic, Resolvent, Sedative, Stimulant, Stomachic, Sudorific, Tonic, Vermifuge, Vulnerary.

PRECAUTIONS: Since it is a very potent oil, low dosage may be advisable though many Aromatherapists avoid using it altogether. Certainly people suffering from epilepsy and high blood pressure should stay clear of it. Not to be used during pregnancy.

MIND: A powerful effect on the mind – gives a feeling of alertness and clarity. Apparently has the ability to release emotional pain by bringing deep feelings into focus. Said to cure grief by clearing the spleen.

BODY: A regulating effect on the circulatory system seems to do a good job in raising low blood pressure. A good tonic to the body when in a weakened condition and its stimulating properties make it useful in convalescence.

Very effective on respiratory problems and viral infections such as colds, coughs, sore throats, influenza, bronchitis and asthma. Helps to clear the lungs and eases tightness in the chest. It fluidifies mucous and relieves bronchial spasm.

A tonic to the digestion and acts as a mild laxative, relieves stomach cramp and expels wind and is said to get rid of worms. Helps restore appetite and aids digestion of fats.

Beneficial to the menstrual cycle particularly with water retention during periods and effective against amenorrhoea and leucorrhoea.

Could give some relief from rheumatism, arthritis and gout.

EFFECT ON SKIN: Has a healing effect on the skin by helping to form scars and disperse bruises. Problem conditions such as dermatitis and eczema may also respond well to this oil.

BLENDS: Angelica, Celery, Fennel, Lavender, Melissa, Orange, Rosemary, Tangerine.

IMMORTELLE

Plant/Part	:	Shrub/Flowers
Latin Name	:	Helichrysum angustifolium
Family	:	Compositae
Note	:	Base
Planet	:	?
Extraction	:	Distillation/Solvent Extraction

AROMA: Strongly woody with a hint of spice.

FEATURES: A wild growing plant, also known to us as 'Italian Everlasting'. It has dark yellow flowers and silver-green pepper scented leaves, the stems reaching to about two feet. It does however, appear in many varieties. Europe, principally Italy, France and Yugoslavia gives us the essential oil. High quality oil is achieved if distillation occurs within 24 hours of harvesting, the younger plants yield greater quantities.

HISTORY & MYTH: Dalmatia began production of Immortelle in 1908. Helichrysum stoechas, another species, shares similar chemical properties and the two were often distilled together. The use of solvents obtains an absolute and much of the work is carried out in the Grasse region of France. Very popular in dried flower decorations.

CHEMICAL CONSTITUENTS: Geraniol, Linalool, Nerol (Alcohols), Neryl acetate (Ester), Pinene (Terpene).

PROPERTIES: Antiphlogistic, Antispasmodic, Antiviral, Astringent, Bacteriacide, Cholagogue, Diuretic, Emollient, Expectorant, Cytophylactic, Fungicide, Hepatic, Sedative, Splenetic.

PRECAUTIONS: ?

MIND: Seems to lessen the effects of shock, fears and phobias and said to relieve depression as well.

BODY: A rejuvenating oil promoting cell growth, helping to rebuild tissues and energise the organs, also improving the general flow of the meridians – the energy channels running through the body.

Clears the body of candida apparently, which often thrives when vitality is low. Since it gives a boost to the immune system, will therefore help to keep such allergies and infections at bay. Also said to regulate blood pressure.

A general aid to the respiratory system soothing feverish colds, influenza, bronchitis, coughs and asthma. Helps to remove mucous from the lungs and induces relaxation and sleep.

Effective aid to the organs of digestion, reducing liver and spleen congestion, dealing with gall bladder disorders and regulating pancreas and bile secretion.

Said to ease the discomfort of rheumatism and general aches and pains. May also relieve persistent headaches and migraine.

Reputedly has a beneficial action on cystitis and herpes simplex.

EFFECT ON SKIN: On a par with Lavender with regard to cell regenerating qualities but probably does not have such strong psychological features. Assists in healing scars, acne, dermatitis, boils and abscesses – a blend with Bergamot, Lavender and Yarrow claims to treat psoriasis. Athletes foot and ringworm seem to respond to its fungicidal properties.

BLENDS: Bergamot, Chamomile, Geranium, Frankincense, lavender, Mandarin, Orange, Petitgrain, Rose, Rosewood, Yarrow.

JASMINE

Plant/Part	:	Tree/Flowers
Latin Name	:	Jasminum grandiflorum
Family	:	Jasminaceae
Note	:	Middle to Base
Planet	:	Jupiter
Extraction	:	Enfleurage/Solvent Extraction

AROMA: Sweet, flowery and exotic – slightly heady.

FEATURES: The delicate white flowers of this climbing tree are picked at night when the aroma is most intense. Jasmine grows to about twenty feet and originates from Iran and northern India. Now grown in Algeria, Morocco, Egypt and Italy as well as France which apparently produces the best oil. The extraction process is a delicate one and demands great skill. Huge quantities are needed to produce the oil, making it very expensive and so subject to adulteration.

HISTORY & MYTH: The 'king of flower oils' has long been used in love potions so powerful was its reputation as an aphrodisiac. Fortuitous it was therefore, that treating gonorrhoea, as well as prostate problems, was also credited to its healing powers! It is widely used for scenting ointments in India as well as for ceremonial purposes. Guests are often decked in bracelets and necklaces made of the flowers.

In Turkey the wood is used in making rope stems and Jasmine tea is a favourite beverage in China. The flowers are a popular garnish in Indonesian cooking and we have to thank the conquering Moors for bringing the plant to Spain. Its extensive use as an ingredient of perfumes continues unabated.

CHEMICAL CONSTITUENTS: Benzyl, Farnesol, Geranoil, Nerol, Terpineol (Alcohols), Linalyl acetate, Methyl anthranilate (Esters), Jasmone (Ketone), Eugenol (Phenol).

PROPERTIES: Antidepressant, Antiseptic, Antispasmodic, Aphrodisiac, Emollient, Galactagogue, Parturient, Sedative, Uterine.

PRECAUTIONS: Not to be used in pregnancy until about to give birth – will then help to ease labour. Its overuse could disturb the bodily fluids especially phlegm and the 'narcotic' like properties may impede concentration. Certainly the powerful aroma indicates low dosage.

MIND: Valuable remedy for severe depression. It is calming to the nerves and warming to the emotions, producing positive feelings of confidence. A boon to people in the 'helping professions' – restoring energy and generally revitalising.

BODY: Perhaps the most valued oil in childbirth. It hastens delivery by strengthening contractions yet relieving pain at the same time. A superb hormone balancer and effective in post-natal depression. Possibly helps to establish a deep bond between mother and child and promotes flow of breast milk.

It also relieves spasm in the uterus, soothes menstrual pain and helpful with vaginal infections generally.

The importance of Jasmine on the male reproductive system is linked to its reputation for increasing the number of spermatozoa, thus reducing infertility. Its deeply relaxing nature may be responsible for its renowned influence over sexual problems such as impotence, premature ejaculation as well as frigidity.

Jasmine is also a boon to the respiratory system. It helps to regulate and deepen breathing by relieving spasm of the bronchi as well as having a calming action on irritating coughs. Said to ease hoarseness as well.

Reputedly loosens up stiff limbs too.

EFFECT ON SKIN: A luxurious but highly effective balm and tonic for dry and sensitive skin though generally beneficial to all types. A blend with Mandarin and Lavender increases skin elasticity and is often used to soften stretch marks and scarring.

BLENDS: Bergamot, Frankincense, Geranium, Guaiacwood, Immortelle, Orange, Mandarin, Melissa, Neroli, Palmarosa, Rose, Rosewood, Sandalwood.

JUNIPER

Plant/Part	:	Bush/Berries
Latin Name	:	Juniperus communis
Family	:	Cupressaceae
Note	:	Middle
Planet	:	Sun
Extraction	:	Distillation

AROMA: Clear, refreshing and slightly woody.

FEATURES: An evergreen shrub and though cultivated to a height of six feet, it spurts to another thirty in the Scandinavian wild. Juniper thrives easily in arctic conditions though it is of course found in many parts of the world. It has a reddish stem, with needle like leaves, supporting small yellow flowers with blue/black berries. Oil obtained from Hungary, France, Italy, Yugoslavia and Canada.

HISTORY & MYTH: Juniper has played a major medicinal role in many contagious diseases such as cholera and typhoid fever. It guarded against the plague in Tibet and the medics of Greece, Rome and Arabia valued its antiseptic properties. In Mongolia, it was given to women at the onset of labour. The 15th and 16th century herbalists praised it highly not only for its effect on the plague but also as a cure for bites. Interestingly enough, the Celtic 'Juneprus' means acrid or biting!

   Juniper and Rosemary twigs were burnt for a long time in French hospitals to clear the air and it was looked upon as a cure-all in Yugoslavia. Once thought to alleviate diabetes. Its ability to replenish tired spirits is inferred in the Bible when the exhausted Elijah slept under a Juniper tree, 1 Kings 19: 4 and 5. And of course, it is famous as an ingredient of gin.

CHEMICAL CONSTITUENTS: Borneol, Terpineol (Alcohols), Cadinene, Cedrene (Sesquiterpenes), Camphene, Mercene, Pinene, Sabinene (Terpenes).

PROPERTIES: Antiseptic, Antirheumatic, Antispasmodic, Aphrodisiac, Astringent, Carminative, Cicatrisant, Depurative, Detoxicant, Disinfectant, Diuretic, Emmenagogue, Nervine, Insecticide, Parturient, Rubefacient, Stimulating, Stomachic, Sudorific, Tonic, Vulnerary.

PRECAUTIONS: Prolonged use may overstimulate the kidneys. Certainly should be avoided in cases of severe kidney disease or other inflammatory conditions. An emmenagogue so best avoided during pregnancy.

MIND: Clears, stimulates and strengthens the nerves. It purifies the atmosphere and supports the spirit in challenging situations. A boon perhaps to people in the 'helping' professions.

BODY: It is a very effective diuretic and antiseptic of the genito-urinary tract, valuable in cystitis, strangury (inability to pass urine) and kidney stones. Helpful in relieving urine when the prostate gland is enlarged. Cellulitis, dropsy and fluid retention could also be set to rights.

Well known for its detoxifying character, driving out toxins particularly when too much alcohol and rich food has been imbibed. Clears mucous from the intestines and could be effective against piles. Generally beneficial to the digestive system, regulating appetite and may be helpful for obesity. A tonic to the liver, has been known to help cirrhosis.

May also stimulate the body when feeling very drowsy and sleepy which could be an indication of waste overload. A foot bath with Juniper could relieve some of the congestion. Its ability to throw off poisons by purifying the blood, makes it valuable where disease-carrying insects abound.

Helps to eliminate uric acid and could be beneficial in cases of arthritis as well as rheumatism, gout and sciatica. Generally strengthens the limbs and of assistance when there is difficult and stiff movement relieving pain in the process.

Also works well on the menstrual cycle, regulating periods and easing painful cramps. Said to help with safe delivery in childbirth.

EFFECT ON SKIN: A tonic for oily and congested skins and for seborrhoea of the scalp. Its purifying properties may ease acne, blocked pores, dermatitis, weeping eczema, psoriasis and swellings.

BLENDS: Benzoin, Bergamot, Cypress, Frankincense, Geranium, Grapefruit, Orange, Lemongrass, Lime, Melissa, Rosemary, Sandalwood.

LAVANDIN

Plant/Part	:	Herb/Flowering tops
Latin Name	:	Lavandula flagrans
Family	:	Labiatae
Note	:	Top
Planet	:	Mercury
Extraction	:	Distillation

AROMA: Clear, sweet and penetrating – similar to Lavender.

FEATURES: True Lavender and Spike produce this European hybrid with just a little help from the pollinating bees. Grown extensively in France between the lower regions of Spike and high elevations of Lavender. The blue/grey flowers are bigger and tougher than the two other species though with less healing powers, or so it is claimed.

HISTORY & MYTH: Since it is hardier than the other two species, the yield of oil is greater overall. However, it was not exported as an oil in its own right initially and was principally used to top up the more fragile Lavender. Since World War Two Lavandin production has increased and is now exported for use in the soap trade and perfumery.

CHEMICAL CONSTITUENTS: Lavandulol, Linalool, Terpineol (Alcohols), Linalyl acetate (Ester), Camphor, Cineole (Ketones), Caryophyllene (Sesquiterpene), Camphene, Dipentene, Limonene, Ocimene, Terpinene (Terpenes).

PROPERTIES: Antidepressant, Analgesic, Antiseptic, Cicatrisant, Expectorant, Nervine, Vulnerary.

PRECAUTIONS: In some ways has similar uses to Lavender though is much less relaxing. Not really suitable for conditions needing a sedative action.

MIND: A refreshing note to a tired mind.

BODY: Especially good for aches and pains and muscle stiffness. May also help with rheumatic discomfort and stiff joints.
   Beneficial to the respiratory tract in particular coughs, colds and

influenza. Certainly eases breathing when lungs and sinuses are choked with phlegm.

EFFECT ON SKIN: Its cicatrisant properties useful in helping wounds to heal and said to have some effect on dermatitis and scabies.

BLENDS: Bergamot, Chamomile, Citronella, Clary Sage, Geranium, Immortelle, Jasmine, Lemon, Orange.

LAVENDER

Plant/Part	:	Shrub/Flowers
Latin Name	:	Lavendula officinalis
Family	:	Labiatae
Note	:	Middle
Planet	:	Mercury
Extraction	:	Distillation

AROMA: Floral, light and clear with woody undertones.

FEATURES: There are quite a few varieties of this lovely plant which grows wild in the Mediterranean – L. Officinalis is said to be the most odorous. Perched on long stems, the tiny purple-blue flowers are covered with star shaped hairs and the narrow leaves are grey/green. Lavender is extensively cultivated in England, France and Yugoslavia.

HISTORY & MYTH: One of the most popular essential oils in Aroma-therapy and used in healing since time immemorial. For centuries, Lavender bags were placed in linen drawers to keep moths and insects at bay – its insecticidal properties being most pronounced. Also revered for its antiseptic quality by the Romans who used it to bathe and cleanse their wounds and indeed the Latin 'lavare' means 'to wash'. Once said to cure milder forms of epilepsy.

  Lavender water was popular in the Elizabethan and Stuart age, and was the favourite perfume of Queen Maria Henrietta, wife to King Charles 1st. English Lavender was grown for a long time around Mitchum in Surrey, though is now cultivated extensively in Norfolk. Its wonderful skin healing properties were discovered quite accidentally, by the French chemist Gattefosse early this century. Imparts an unusual flavour to some Moroccan and French dishes.

CHEMICAL CONSTITUENTS: Borneol, Geraniol, Lavandulol, Linalool (Alcohols), Geranyl acetate, Lavandulyl acetate, Linalyl acetate (Ester), Cineole (Ketone), Caryophyllene (Sesquiterpene), Limonene, Pinene (Terpenes).

PROPERTIES: Analgesic, Anticonvulsive, Antidepressant, Antiphlogistic, Antirheumatic, Antiseptic, Antispasmodic, Antiviral, Bacteriacide, Carminative, Cholagogue, Cicatrisant, Cordial, Cytophylactic, Decongestant,

Deodorant, Detoxicant, Diuretic, Emmenagogue, Fungicide, Hypotensive, Nervine, Restorative, Sedative, Splenetic, Sudorific, Vulnerary.

PRECAUTIONS: Some people with low blood pressure may feel a bit dull and drowsy after using this oil. It is an emmenagogue too, so best avoided in the early months of pregnancy.

MIND: Rudolf Steiner suggested that Lavender stabilises the Physical, Etheric and Astral bodies which indicates a positive effect on psychological disorders. It appears to cleanse and soothe the Spirit relieving anger and exhaustion, resulting in a calmer approach to life. Its balancing action on the Central Nervous System may well be valuable in manic-depressive states.

BODY: Has a sedative action on the heart and will help to bring down high blood pressure and calm palpitations. Long known as giving effective relief from insomnia.

Its pain relieving qualities deal effectively with muscular spasm and in this regard may be good for sprains, strains, and sharp rheumatic pains. A blend with Marjoram enhances the effect.

Beneficial to the respiratory system and deals with such problems as bronchitis, asthma, catarrh, colds, laryngitis and throat infections. An aid in relieving the effects of tuberculosis and with its anti-viral properties keeps infection down.

Useful with menstrual problems such as scanty or painful periods and leuchorrhoea. May be helpful in childbirth, relieving pain and speeding delivery. Massage of the lower back helps to expel afterbirth.

Said to clear the spleen (apparently the seat of anger) and the liver. It increases gastric secretion and could be of use in nausea, vomiting, colic and flatulence. Stimulates bile production which helps digestion of fats.

Renowned as an insecticide so keeps moths and insects at bay. Also said to cleanse dog bites and purify the air.

EFFECT ON SKIN: Valuable for most skin conditions since it promotes growth of new cells and exerts a balancing action on sebum. It has a pronounced healing effect on burns and sunburn and helpful in cases of acne, eczema and psoriasis. Also said to heal abscesses, boils and carbuncles as well as minimise fungal growths, swellings, scarring and gangrenous wounds. An effective hair tonic too and may be of service in cases of alopecia.

BLENDS: Bay, Bergamot, Chamomile, Citronella, Clary Sage, Geranium, Jasmine, Lemon, Mandarin, Nutmeg, Orange, Patchouli, Pine, Thyme, Rosemary.

LAVENDER SPIKE

Plant/Part	:	Shrub/Flowering tops
Latin Name	:	Lavendula spica/latifolia
Family	:	Labiatae
Note	:	Top
Planet	:	Mercury
Extraction	:	Distillation

AROMA: Similar to Lavender though clearer and fresher.

FEATURES: A more robust plant than true Lavender and somewhat taller. It has blue/grey flowers and enjoys growing by the sea. The essential oil is often obtained from Spain, Italy and France.

HISTORY & MYTH: Sometimes referred to as 'male lavender' due to its more 'aggressive' properties – no sexism intended! Being more camphoraceous and harsher it is used to perfume cheaper goods and is often employed in the varnishing industry. It thrived in a wild state all over Spain and workers would stoop for hours cutting Spike for distillation. Labour was cheap since Spain was a mainly rural population up to the Civil War.

However, since 1936 the output decreased and France took over production. Adulteration of Spike with Sage oil was once all too frequent – due to the unreasonable price demands on the part of buyers it seems. Has been used for veterinary purposes possibly to cleanse wounds.

CHEMICAL CONSTITUENTS: Camphor, Cineole (Ketones), Camphene (Terpene), Borneol, Linalool (Alcohols).

PROPERTIES: Analgesic, Antidepressant, Antiseptic, Antiviral, Decongestant, Insecticide.

PRECAUTIONS: Its gentler cousin is emmenagogic, so just to be on the safe side, perhaps best avoided in pregnancy. Large amounts may over-activate the central nervous system which could produce palpitations.

MIND: A cerebro-spinal tranquilliser, helps to clear a stuffy head makes the senses calmer yet more alert.

BODY: Particularly effective on respiratory complaints such as bronchitis and laryngitis. Eases breathing and clears the head, relieving headaches linked to catarrh. Could well build up immunity to further viral attacks.

Its analgesic properties tend to lessen muscular and rheumatic pain promoting relaxation of the nerve fibres. It appears that its general balancing qualities are able to balance excess heat or cold in the muscles sometimes evident after injury.

Relieves painful stings and insect bites.

EFFECT ON SKIN: May help with the formation of scar tissue and could well have some fungicidal properties relieving ringworm and athletes foot.

BLENDS: Bergamot, Chamomile, Geranium, Guaiacwood, Immortelle, Jasmine, Lemon, Orange.

LEMON

Plant/Part	:	Fruit/Peel
Latin Name	:	Citrus limonum
Family	:	Rutaceae
Note	:	Top
Planet	:	Sun
Extraction	:	Expression/Distillation

AROMA: A citrus fragrance – fresh and sharp.

FEATURES: A small thorny evergreen tree, native to India though often grown in southern Europe, Florida and California. It has irregular branches, shiny oval leaves with white/pink strongly perfumed flowers. There are several varieties of Lemon which differ in rind thickness and percentage of juice, the green unripe fruits being a richer source of essential oil. Hand expression still yields a better quality oil than more recent methods of distillation.

HISTORY & MYTH: Long valued as an antiseptic against bites from disease carrying insects – once thought to be useful in treating malaria. Its hypotensive effect on arteriosclerosis was recognised too. The Egyptians saw it as an antidote to meat and fish poisoning and typhoid epidemics.

Lemon is derived from the Arab 'laimun' and Persian 'limun' referring to citrus fruits. The holy wars of the early middle ages were a source of rich treasures brought back to Europe by the Crusadors, amongst which was the humble Lemon. Italy became an important Lemon producing country latterly followed by California. The fresh fruit has long been used for its Vitamin C content thought once to be a tonic to the endocrine glands. A popular flavouring agent in foods and perfumes.

CHEMICAL CONSTITUENTS: Linalool (Alcohol), Citral, Citronellal (Aldehydes), Cadinene (Sesquiterpene), Bisabolene, Camphene, Dipentene, Limonene, Pinene, Phellandrene (Terpenes).

PROPERTIES: Antiacid, Antisclerotic, Antiscorbutic, Antineuralgic, Antirheumatic, Antipruritic, Antiseptic, Astringent, Bactericide, Carminative, Cicatrisant, Depurative, Diuretic, Emollient, Escharotic, Febrifuge, Haemostatic, Hepatic, Hypoglycemiant, Hypotensive, Insecticide, Laxative, Stomachic, Tonic, Vermifuge.

PRECAUTIONS: May irritate sensitive skin.

MIND: Refreshing and cooling when feeling hot and bothered, helping to produce clarity of thought.

BODY: A superb tonic to the circulatory system, liquefying the blood and aiding flow thus easing pressure on varicose veins. An effective heart tonic and often used in bringing down high blood pressure. Restores vitality to red corpuscles easing anaemic conditions. At the same time stimulates the white corpuscles thereby invigorating the immune system and aiding the body to fight infectious disease.

Said to be helpful for nosebleeds and stems external bleeding generally.

Its antiseptic nature relieves sore throats, coughs, colds and influenza particularly when accompanied by feverish conditions as it reduces high temperatures. Seems to ease painful cold sores and herpes.

Improves the functioning of the digestive system, counteracts acidity in the body and makes the stomach more alkaline. Apparently helps with pancreatic secretions and has been used to treat diabetes. Has a decongestant action on the kidneys and liver and a cleansing action on the body generally. Could be helpful with constipation and cellulite.

Said to relieve headaches and migraine as well as neuralgic pains, rheumatism and arthritis.

Will soothe insect bites and stings.

EFFECT ON SKIN: Brightens pale and dull complexions by removing dead skin cells. It smooths out broken capillaries and has an effective cleansing action on greasy skin and hair. A popular remedy for removing corns, warts and verrucas. Also has a softening effect on scar tissue and guards against brittle nails.

BLENDS: Benzoin, Cardamom, Chamomile, Eucalyptus, Fennel, Frankincense, Ginger, Juniper, Lavender, Linden, Blossom Neroli, Rose, Sandalwood, Ylang Ylang.

LEMONGRASS

Plant/Part	:	Grass/Leaves
Latin Name	:	Cymbopogon citratus/ flexuosus
Family	:	Gramineae
Note	:	Top
Planet	:	?
Extraction	:	Distillation

AROMA: Strong, sweet and lemony.

FEATURES: This rather sharp yet lovely essential oil is distilled from two species of cultivated fresh grass. The wild variety would be too costly to gather. Originally from India, it also grows in other tropical areas such as Brazil, West Indies, Sri Lanka and China. Just tips three feet in height.

HISTORY & MYTH: A favourite oil in India for hundreds of years and known locally as 'choomana poolu' which refers to the plant's red grass stems. Otherwise known as 'Indian Verbena' or 'Indian Melissa Oil' and was thought to be helpful in bringing down fevers, reducing infectious diseases and arresting the development of tumours.

India was the main supplier until the Second World War after which production was taken over by the West Indies which now produces the finer quality oil apparently. The East Indian variety is C. Flexuosus and West Indian, C. Citratus. A good quality oil is also obtained from the USA. Exposure to air and light lowers the citral content of the oil, which is valuable as an ingredient of cosmetics and perfumes as well as detergents and soaps.

CHEMICAL CONSTITUENTS: Farnesol, Geraniol, Nerol (Alcohols), Citral, Citronellal (Aldehydes), Limonene, Myrcene (Terpenes).

PROPERTIES: Antidepressant, Antiseptic, Bacteriacide, Carminative, Deodorant, Digestive, Diuretic, Fungicide, Galactagogue, Insecticide, Prophylactic, Stimulant, Tonic.

PRECAUTIONS: A rather harsh essential oil and could irritate sensitive skins. Low dosage is best.

MIND: Stimulating, reviving, and energising, useful in states of exhaustion. Lifts the spirits and gets things moving again.

BODY: A revitalising action makes it a good tonic for the body. It gives a boost to the parasympathetic nerves which aids recovery from illness stimulating glandular secretions and the muscles in digestion. Encourages appetite and could be helpful with colitis, indigestion and gastro-enteritis.

Its strong antiseptic action prevents the spread of contagious diseases, useful particularly with respiratory infections such as sore throats, laryngitis and fevers.

Excellent for aching muscles, relieves pain and makes them more supple since it helps to eliminate lactic acid and stimulates circulation. Its toning effect on muscles may help with loose skin due to dieting or lack of exercise. Seems to relieve tired legs, especially after standing for long periods of time.

Its invigorating action on the body mitigates some of the symptoms of jet lag, clearing headaches and relieving fatigue.

Useful in keeping insects away and ridding animals of pests and fleas. Its deodorant action keeps them nice smelling too.

Also aids the flow of breast milk in nursing mothers.

EFFECT ON SKIN: Gives good tone to the skin and may be effective in open pores. Reputedly able to clear acne and balance oily conditions. Athletes foot and other fungal infections could respond favourably.

BLENDS: Basil, Cedarwood, Coriander, Geranium, Jasmine, Lavender, Neroli, Niaouli, Palmarosa, Rosemary, Ti-Tree, Yarrow.

LIME

Plant/Part	:	Fruit/Peel
Latin Name	:	Citrus medica/aurantifolia
Family	:	Rutaceae
Note	:	Top
Planet	:	Sun
Extraction	:	Expression and Distillation

AROMA: Rather sharp and bitter-sweet.

FEATURES: Originally from Asia, the Lime fruit is cultivated in many warm countries notably Italy, the West Indies and the Americas. It resembles Lemon in appearance but tends to be more greenish and globular instead of oval. Though there are many varieties of Lime, it usually measures about two inches in diameter. The expressed oil is much lighter and apparently has a sweeter fragrance.

HISTORY & MYTH: Apparently introduced into Europe by the Moors and subsequently brought to America by the Spanish and Portuguese explorers around 16th century. Ships bearing Lime were called 'lime juicers', since crews depended upon it to prevent scurvy – a dietary deficiency causing general weakness. Lime has since been a good source of Vitamin C.

The juice and fruit industry originated in the West Indies around 19th century and the oil has been used to flavour ginger ale and cola drinks. It is used extensively in the perfume industry. Some sweet Lime oil is available, resembling Bergamot in aroma.

CHEMICAL CONSTITUENTS: Linalool, Terpineol (Alcohols, Citral (Aldehyde), Linalyl acetate (Ester), Bergaptene (Lactone), Limonene, Pinene, Sabinene, Terpinoline (Terpenes).

PROPERTIES: Antiscorbutic, Antiseptic, Antiviral, Aperitif, Astringent, Bacteriacide, Disinfectant, Febrifuge, Haemostatic, Insecticide, Restorative, Tonic.

PRECAUTIONS: May cause photosensitivity in presence of strong sunlight and possibility of irritating sensitive skin.

MIND: Very activating and stimulating especially where there is apathy, anxiety and depression. Refreshing and uplifting to a tired mind.

BODY: May help to cool feverish conditions which accompany colds, sore throats and influenza. Eases coughs, congestion of the chest, catarrh and sinusitis. A tonic to the immune system and keeps infection down. Gives back energy after illness.

A digestive stimulant, like most citrus oils, and may be useful to sufferers from anorexia since it encourages appetite by stimulating the digestive secretions.

Said to treat the effects of alcoholism possibly because of its disinfecting and restorative properties.

Reputedly helpful with rheumatic pain.

EFFECT ON SKIN: Its astringent, toning and refreshing action seems to clear greasy skin. Also said to stem bleeding from cuts and wounds.

BLENDS: Angelica, Bergamot, Geranium, Linden Blossom, Lavender, Neroli, Nutmeg, Palmarosa, Rose, Violet, Ylang Ylang.

LINDEN BLOSSOM

Plant/Part	:	Tree/Flowers
Latin Name	:	Tilia europaea
Family	:	Tiliaceae
Note	:	Base
Planet	:	Jupiter or Venus
Extraction	:	Enfleurage

AROMA: Sweet, deep and slightly spicy, rather long lasting.

FEATURES: The Europaea, said to be a cross between T. platyphyllos and T. cordata, is a familiar sight along many European and English avenues. It reaches to about a hundred feet and is also known as 'Lime Tree'. A dull grey bark supports wide branches with dark green serrated leaves above and light green below. The abundant nectar contained in the pendulous white flowers sends bees into paroxysms of delight.

HISTORY & MYTH: An association with witchcraft went hand in hand with the Blossom's reputation in curing epilepsy and paralysis. The ancient Germanic races ignored the potential ill omens and made the Linden Tree a symbol of their nation. The Romans were a little more practical and boiled the inner bark with meat to make it less salty. Linden blossoms have often been mixed with hops to induce sleep, indeed a popular drink in France called 'Tilleuil' is thought to relieve insomnia and indigestion.

At one time Lime charcoal from the wood was mixed with water to assimilate stomach poisons. It was also thought to reduce sweating and was once used in festering wounds and cancerous growths. The name 'Tilia' may be derived from the old 'Ptilon', meaning 'feather' indicating the feathery appearance of the leaves. The master carver, Grinling Gibbons favoured the wood for carving. Unfortunately, it seems the natural flower oil is hard to come by since it can be successfully reproduced commercially.

CHEMICAL CONSTITUENTS: Farnesol (Alcohol).

PROPERTIES: Antispasmodic, Astringent, Bechic, Cephalic, Decongestant, Diuretic, Emollient, Hypotensive, Nervine, Sedative, Sudorific, Tonic.

PRECAUTIONS: The aroma might be a little too 'heady' for some people and there's also a chance of causing allergy to sensitive skins.

MIND: A very relaxing oil promoting sound sleep.

BODY: An excellent tonic for the nervous system, helpful with headaches, migraine, neuralgia and vertigo. Also said to be effective against high blood pressure resulting from nervous tension. Its purifying and thinning action on the blood could help with chronic circulatory diseases, helping to clear high cholesterol levels and apparently has a beneficial action on anaemia.

Useful in chronic catarrhal conditions, helps to bring down feverish colds by increasing perspiration yet said to decrease night sweats. Effective against respiratory illnesses generally, i.e. influenza, pleurisy and bronchitis. Gets rid of that stuffed up feeling, helps to clear air passages, facilitates breathing and eases coughs.

Its diuretic action beneficial on kidney disorders clearing any mucous. A tonic and detoxifying effect on the liver could help relieve hepatitis. Seems to be effective on disorders of the stomach, indigestion and diarrhoea. Could help to banish mouth ulcers.

Clears excess urea and may be effective against rheumatism, gout as well as sciatica.

Apparently strengthens the muscles of the eyes but should not of course, be used directly on them.

EFFECT ON SKIN: Its soothing, softening and toning action is said to keep wrinkles at bay! Also boasts a reputation for dealing with blemishes, freckles and burns as well as having a tonic effect on the scalp encouraging hair growth.

BLENDS: Benzoin, Citronella, Ginger, Grapefruit, Jasmine, Lavender, Neroli, Palmarosa, Rose, Verbena, Violet, Ylang Ylang.

LITSEA CUBEBA

Plant/Part	:	Tree/Fruit
Latin Name	:	Litsea cubeba
Family	:	Lauraceae
Note	:	Top
Planet	:	?
Extraction	:	Distillation

AROMA: A sweet citrus and fruity fragrance with floral undertones.

FEATURES: A small tree from asia with spicy fruits and fragrant leaves and flowers. Produced in China and Malaysia and known there as 'Chinese Pepper' and 'May Chang' not to mention 'Mountain Spice Tree' as well.

HISTORY & MYTH: This celebrated tree of Eastern origin has only recently become well known in the Western world. It was in the 1950's that the essential oil was first distilled from the pepper-like fruits and began to compete in popularity with Lemongrass oil which tends to have more 'fatty' notes. The citral content of the two oils is almost identical though Lemongrass has a more lingering quality.

Besides being used as a flavouring agent in Chinese cooking, it was also used to treat cancer tumours since it was thought to have a carcinostatic quality. These days Litsea Cubeba is widely used as an ingredient of soaps, perfumes and deodorants.

CHEMICAL CONSTITUENTS: Geranoil, Linalool (Alcohol), Citral, Citronellal (Aldehydes), Linalyl acetate (Ester), Cineole (Ketone), Cadinene (Sesquiterpene), Limonene, Sabinene (Terpenes).

PRECAUTIONS: A rather strong aroma so care should be taken with dosage.

PROPERTIES: Antidepressant, Antiseptic, Astringent, Bacteriacide, Carminative, Galactagogue, Insecticide, Stimulant, Tonic.

MIND: Very uplifting and stimulating – seems to create a 'sunny' atmosphere.

BODY: May well have a stimulating and revitalising effect on the body being a tonic to the heart and respiratory system. Seems to be particularly useful in 'low energy' states.

Said to be a bronchodilator and may be helpful in cases of bronchitis and asthma. Some reports state that it has a beneficial effect on coronary heart disease.

May well be a digestive stimulant and could relieve flatulence, nausea and encourage appetite. Said to ease oral thrush as well as proving useful with lactation difficulties.

EFFECT ON SKIN: Tonic and astringent properties encourage a balancing action on oily skin and hair.

BLENDS: Basil, Geranium, Guaiacwood, Jasmine, Lavender, Neroli, Orange, Petitgrain, Rose, Rosemary, Rosewood, Verbena, Ylang Ylang.

MANDARIN

Plant/Part	:	Tree/Peel
Latin Name	:	Citrus madurensis
Family	:	Rutaceae
Note	:	Top to Middle
Planet	:	?
Extraction	:	Expression

AROMA: Delicate, sweet, tangy with floral undertones.

FEATURES: A prolific producing fruit tree which likes hot and humid climates. Trees growing in more temperate zones however, seem to produce larger amounts of oil and semi-ripe fruit has the greatest yield. Producing areas include Brazil, Spain, Italy and California. Tangerine which is from the same botanical source, apparently has a weaker aroma or should we say rather more delicate?

HISTORY & MYTH: It seems a little strange that the rulers of China were once called Mandarins when the name is now so much associated with the fruit! This soft, orange fruit was once given to their oriental majesties as a token of respect, hence its name. The last 200 years has seen its popularity grow in Europe where it is extensively cultivated particularly in the Mediterranean region.

The production of oil has also been expanding in America though temporarily halted during the Second World War due to difficulty in importing the Italian fruit. Brazil took over exportation to the USA though it is said that the Italian essential oil is lighter and of superior quality. Much use is found for Mandarin oil in the world of perfumery and catering.

CHEMICAL CONSTITUENTS: Geraniol (Alcohol), Citral, Citronellal (Aldehydes), Methyl Anthranilate (Ester), Limonene (Terpene).

PROPERTIES: Antispasmodic, Cholagogue, Cytophylactic, Digestive, Emollient, Sedative, Tonic.

PRECAUTIONS: May be phototoxic, so best not to use before going out into strong sunlight.

MIND: Its refreshing aroma has an uplifting quality and often helps to banish depression and anxiety.

BODY: A tonic to the digestion, stimulates appetite, particularly after illness or loss of hunger due to depression. Seems to have a stimulating effect on the liver, helping to regulate metabolic processes and aids in the secretion of bile and breaking down fats. At the same time it is calming to the intestines and good for expelling gas.

Has a reputation for being a mild oil and is often used on children (in smaller dosage) and pregnant women – anyone who is feeling a little fragile in fact. Seems to have a revitalising and strengthening effect.

Its cheering action is sometimes used as part of a blend to ease pre menstrual tension. Possibly has an enhanced effect when blended with other citrus oils.

EFFECT ON SKIN: Often used in combination with Neroli and Lavender to lessen stretch marks and scarring.

BLENDS: Basil, Bergamot, Black Pepper, Coriander, Chamomile, Grapefruit, Lavender, Lemon, Lime, Marjoram, Neroli, Palmarosa, Petitgrain, Rose.

MARJORAM

Plant/Part	:	Herb/Flowering heads/leaves
Latin Name	:	Origanum marjorana
Family	:	Labiatae
Note	:	Middle
Planet	:	Mercury
Extraction	:	Distillation

AROMA: Warm, penetrating and slightly spicy.

FEATURES: There are several varieties of Marjoram though its most familiar to us as a small plant reaching to about ten inches with small oval leaves and white or pink flowers. The sweet Marjoram originates from Libya, Egypt and the Mediterranean region though much of the oil is obtained from France. Wild Marjoram (Thymus mastichina) from Spain is apparently of inferior quality.

HISTORY & MYTH: It was a very popular and common medicinal herb amongst the ancient Greeks. They used it to treat spasm and excess fluid in the tissues and thought it a valuable antidote against poison. Certainly it was seen as a digestive herb. The Greek 'orosganos' meaning 'joy of the mountain' seems quite apt since it was given to newlyweds as a token of good fortune. Yet it was also planted in graveyards to help bring peace to the departed spirit.

In Latin, the 'Marjor' prefix means 'great' attributed to prolonging life. In Stuart times, nosegays contained Marjoram to mask unpleasant smells. There was also a hint of it in aromatic waters, not to mention snuff and pizzas in latter days.

CHEMICAL CONSTITUENTS: Borneol, Terpineol (Alcohols), Camphor (Ketone), Caryophyllene (Sesquiterpene), Pinene, Sabinene, Terpinene (Terpenes).

PROPERTIES: Analgesic, Anaphrodisiac, Antiseptic, Antispasmodic, Carminative, Cephalic, Cordial, Digestive, Emmenagogue, Expectorant, Hypotensive, Laxative, Nervine, Restorative, Sedative, Tonic, Vulnerary.

PRECAUTIONS: Prolonged use can cause drowsiness and best avoided during pregnancy.

MIND: Has a calming effect on the nervous system, relieving anxiety, stress and perhaps deeper psychological traumas. It strengthens the mind and helps to confront issues. May give a feeling of comfort in cases of grief and loneliness since it has warming effect on the emotions. Excellent for hyperactive people.

BODY: A really useful oil, promoting good health in many different ways. Particularly effective in dealing with painful muscles, notably in the lower back area possibly when connected to digestive problems and menstrual disorders.

May also help with rheumatic aches and pains and swollen joints, especially where there is a feeling of cold and stiffness. This action is brought about by its effect on the circulation. It dilates the arteries and capillaries, allowing easier flow of blood, promoting a feeling of well being and warmth. Beneficial as an after-sports rub.

A good tonic to the heart and seems to lower high blood pressure. Its generally relaxing effect is helpful for headaches, migraines and insomnia.

Well known for its soothing effect on the digestion and may help with stomach cramps, indigestion, constipation, flatulence and could aid the body in clearing toxins. Possibly effective against sea-sickness.

Seems to have a beneficial action on chest infections as well as colds, sinusitis, bronchitis and asthma. Helps to clear the head during colds and alleviates that stuffed-up feeling.

Could be useful in regulating the menstrual cycle and relieving painful periods. However, it has a reputation for quelling sexual desire!

EFFECT ON SKIN: Valuable in clearing bruises since promotes easier flow of blood.

BLENDS: Bergamot, Cedarwood, Chamomile, Cypress, Lavender, Mandarin, Orange, Nutmeg, Rosemary, Rosewood, Ylang Ylang.

MELISSA

Plant/Part	:	Herb/leaves and flowers
Latin Name	:	Melissa officinalis
Family	:	Labiatae
Note	:	Middle
Planet	:	Jupiter
Extraction	:	Distillation

AROMA: Sweet and lemon-like with floral undertones.

FEATURES: A Mediterranean plant with France producing most of the oil. Melissa favours soil containing iron which may account for its reputed anti-anaemic action. It grows to about two feet and has small, slightly hairy, wrinkled, serrated leaves. The yellowish flowers are attractive to bees and Melissa is the Greek word for honey-bee.

HISTORY & MYTH: Apparently bees fed honey to the infant Jupiter which his mother Rhea hid from her husband Chronus. Indeed honey produced from Melissa is said to be delicious – a godlike nectar perhaps! Paracelsus, a famous Swiss medic, called Melissa 'The Elixir of Life' due to its calming action on the heart no doubt. Famed for its rejuvenating properties and has a reputation as a 'cure all'. The plant has been in long medicinal use and was popular in the Middle East as a cordial.

Also known as 'Lemon Balm', an abbreviation of balsam as well as the Hebrew 'Bal-Smin' meaning 'Chief of Oils'. It was introduced into Britain by the Romans and has remained a popular herb since that time. In the 14th century, it was included in a tonic water made by French Carmelite nuns. During the Elizabethan age, the leaves found a place in wine making and latterly in furniture polish. Often adulterated and true Melissa is expensive. Sometimes referred to as 'Citronelle' in France.

CHEMICAL CONSTITUENTS: Citronellic (Acid), Citronellol, Geraniol, Linalool (Alcohols), Citral, Citronellal (Aldehydes), Geranyl acetate (Ester), Caryophyllene (Sesquiterpene).

PRECAUTIONS: As it helps to regulate menstruation, best avoided in pregnancy. May also irritate sensitive skin.

PROPERTIES: Antiallergenic, Antidepressant, Antispasmodic, Carminative, Cordial, Digestive, Febrifuge, Hypotensive, Nervine, Sedative, Stomachic, Sudorific, Tonic, Uterine.

MIND: Seems to have a calming yet uplifting effect on the emotions dealing with hyper-sensitive states. Said to remove 'blocks' and very soothing in cases of shock, panic and hysteria. Possibly gives comfort to the bereaved, helping to face loss and instilling a positive outlook.

BODY: Its calming effect is a balm to the circulatory system easing high blood pressure, slowing down heartbeat and helpful where the system has been over-stimulated. A good tonic for the heart generally, useful in spasm and fatigue.

Seems to have an affinity with the female reproductive system, regulating periods and promoting a soothing and relaxing action on painful menstruation. Its tonic effect on the uterus could be of benefit in some cases of conception difficulties.

May also settle the stomach and digestion including nausea, flatulence, vomiting, dyspepsia and dysentery.

Could help with colds and has a cooling effect on fevers. Seems to ease migraine and headaches associated with colds.

Effective as an insect repellant and has a soothing action on stings.

A reputation for counteracting allergies may prove helpful for asthma sufferers – seems to have a calming action on rapid breathing.

EFFECT ON SKIN: Checks blood flow in wounds apparently and may have some effect on fungal infections as well as eczema. Said to clear greasy hair and counteract baldness.

BLENDS: Basil, Bay, Chamomile, Frankincense, Geranium, Ginger, Guaiacwood, Jasmine, Juniper, Lavender, Marjoram, Neroli, Rose, Rosemary, Violet, Ylang Ylang.

MYRRH

Plant/Part	:	Bush/Stem/Branches
Latin Name	:	Commiphora myrrha
Family	:	Burseraceae
Note	:	Base
Planet	:	Sun
Extaction	:	Distillation

AROMA: Smoky, gum-like and slightly musky.

FEATURES: There are many species of this well known shrub which grows to about nine feet. A native of North Africa, Asia, and Somalia, the oil is normally obtained from the Middle East. When the grey bark is cut, the gum resin exudes as a yellowish-white fluid which dries into reddish-brown lumps from which the oil is distilled. Fragments of the gum were also collected from the beards of goats who munched on the tasty leaves!

HISTORY & MYTH: Its widespread use in the ancient world was a testimony to Myrrh's popularity. The Egyptians would burn Myrrh, known as 'phun', at noon every day as part of their sun-worshipping ritual. They also combined it with Coriander and Honey in an unguent for treating herpes. Indeed it had a broad medicinal use. Myrrh was also employed in top grade mummification as well as in cosmetics, especially facial masks.

The Book of Esther talks about its use in the purification of women and when Joseph was sold by his brothers to the Ishmaelite caravan, their camels were carrying gum, balm and Myrrh to Egypt. Greek soldiers took a phial of Myrrh into battle – its antiseptic and anti-inflammatory properties helped stem their bleeding wounds. It was a gift to the infant Jesus (Matthew 2, 11) at his birth and also handed to him on the cross mixed with wine (Mark 15, 23).

CHEMICAL CONSTITUENTS: Myrrholic (Acid), Cinnamic, Cuminic (Aldehydes), Eugenol (Phenol), Cadinene (Sesquiterpene), Pinene, Dipentene, Heerabolene, Limonene (Terpenes).

PROPERTIES: Antiseptic, Antimicrobe, Antiphlogistic, Astringent, Balsamic, Deodorant, Carminative, Disinfectant, Diuretic, Emmenagogue,

Expectorant, Fungicide, Stimulant, Stomachic, Sudorific, Tonic, Uterine, Vulnerary.

PRECAUTIONS: An emmenagogue so best avoided in pregnancy.

MIND: Seems to give a lift to feelings of weakness, apathy and lack of incentive. However, also said to have a cooling effect on heated emotions.

BODY: Principally has a 'drying' action and effective against excessive mucous in the lungs. It is said to work powerfully on pulmonary complaints generally, being cleansing in action and treating such ailments as bronchitis, colds, sore throats, catarrh, pharyngitis and coughs. Supposedly helpful with glandular fever, a virus accompanied by sore throat.

Excellent for all mouth and gum disorders – said to be about the best treatment for ulcers, pyorrhoea, gingivitis and spongy gums. May also help with bad breath due to abnormal gastric fermentations. A tonic to the stomach therefore, stimulating appetite, stemming diarrhoea, easing flatulence, acidity and piles.

Of great benefit to gynaecological problems apparently, dealing with scanty periods, leucorrhoea, thrush and clearing obstructions in the womb.

Said to stimulate white blood corpuscles and invigorate the immune system. Its direct antimicrobe effect helps quick recovery from disease.

EFFECT ON SKIN: Powerful skin preservative properties reputedly check tissue degeneration which might be valuable in cases of gangrene. Its cooling action can help reduce boils, skin ulcers, sores, especially bed sores as well as controlling weeping wounds and chapped, moist skin. May deal effectively with weeping eczema and athletes foot.

BLENDS: Benzoin, Clove, Frankincense, Galbanum, Lavender, Patchouli, Sandalwood.

MYRTLE

Plant/Part	:	Bush/Leaves
Latin Name	:	Myrtus communis
Family	:	Myrtaceae
Note	:	Middle
Planet	:	Venus or Mercury
Extraction	:	Distillation

AROMA: Fresh, slightly sweet and penetrating.

FEATURES: Myrtle was once a wild growing bush found in North Africa and Iran. It is now cultivated throughout the Mediterranean, where together with Rosemary, forms the typical landscape. It is a small evergreen with glossy green/blue leaves, white flowers and black berries. Corsican essential oil was said to be the best at one time, though much is now produced in Morocco, Austria and Tunisia.

HISTORY & MYTH: The Egyptians used Myrtle to ease facial tics and the Romans thought it a panacea for respiratory and urinary problems. The more lyrical Greeks held it to be a symbol of love and immortality. Indeed, its fame as an aphrodisiac was most persistent and was often an ingredient of love potions. A myth goes that Phaedra, wife of Theseus, fell in love with Hippolytus, in the shadow of a Myrtle tree. It was an ingredient of perfumes and spicy wines such as the Roman 'Myrtidanum'. Victors were often crowned with Myrtle leaves at the Olympic games.

It is mentioned in the Bible in connection with peace – Nehemiah 8, 15 and Zecharia 1, 8 and 11. Often included in wedding bouquets and headdresses, it was also dried and used as a dusting powder for babies. Later in the 16th century, Myrtle was thought to be effective against skin cancers. It was also an ingredient of 'angel water' – a skin tonic.

CHEMICAL CONSTITUENTS: Geraniol, Linalool, Myrtenol, Nerol (Alcohols), Myrtenal (Aldehyde), Cineole (Ketone), Camphene, Dipentene, Pinene (Terpenes).

PROPERTIES: Antiseptic, Astringent, Bacteriacide, Carminative, Expectorant, Parasiticide.

PRECAUTIONS: Could possibly irritate mucous membranes with prolonged use.

MIND: May soothe feelings of anger.

BODY: Seems to have a pronounced clearing effect and particularly useful with pulmonary disorders especially when accompanied by night sweats. Indeed, promotes restful sleep due to its sedative nature and perhaps more beneficial at night than the stimulating Eucalyptus which it resembles in action. Both oils are helpful in combatting excessive moisture, bronchial catarrh and clearing sinusitis. Generally effective in keeping infection down.

Also has been noted for its regulating effect on the genito-urinary system, easing such problems as haemorrhoids, diarrhoea and dysentery. Furthermore, its antiseptic properties may help to clear cystitis and urethritis.

Could stem leucorrhoea, help to loosen general congestion of the pelvic organs and said to be an effective tonic to the womb.

Reputedly helps to keep vermin away.

EFFECT ON SKIN: Its antiseptic and astringent qualities seem to have a cleansing action on congested skin. Could therefore be useful in the treatment of acne as well as clearing blemishes generally and bruises particularly. May also alleviate the scaling appearance of psoriasis.

BLENDS: Bergamot, Cardamom, Coriander, Dill, Lavender, Lemon, Lemongrass, Rosewood, Rosemary, Spearmint, Thyme, Ti-Tree.

NEROLI

Plant/Part	:	Orange Tree/Petals
Latin Name	:	Citrus aurantium/vulgaris
Family	:	Rutaceae
Note	:	Middle to Base
Planet	:	Sun
Extraction	:	Enfleurage/Distillation

AROMA: A beautiful floral fragrance and rather haunting.

FEATURES: The orange tree originally came from China though Neroli essential oil is generally obtained from France, Morocco, Portugal and Italy. The white petals from the bitter Seville orange (C. vulgaris) gives us Neroli Bigarade which is said to be the best oil. The sweet orange (C. aurantium) is known as Neroli of Portugal. Some Neroli oil is made from the lemon and mandarin blossom.

HISTORY & MYTH: The name is said to originate from an Italian princess, Anne-Marie, Countess of Neroli, who used the oil as a perfume and to scent her gloves and bathwater. Orange flower petals have long been a feature of wedding bouquets symbolising innocence as well as securing love.

The petals were used extensively in China in making cosmetics and latterly in Victorian times as an ingredient of eau de cologne for the 'vapours' frequently suffered by tight-laced ladies. Orange flower water is a popular cooking medium in many Eastern European dishes. A very expensive oil – it takes a great mass of flowers to make a thimbleful of oil. Orange flower water is often used in skin care cosmetics and as an ingredient of eau de cologne.

CHEMICAL CONSTITUENTS: Phenylacetic (Acid), Nerol, Geraniol, Linalool, Nerolidol, Terpineol (Alcohols), Linalyl acetate, Methyl anthranilate, Neryl acetate (Esters), Jasmone (Ketone), Indole (Nitrogen), Camphene, Limonene (Terpenes).

PROPERTIES: Antidepressant, Antiseptic, Antispasmodic, Aphrodisiac, Bacteriacide, Carminative, Cordial, Cytophylactic, Deodorant, Digestive, Emollient, Sedative, Tonic.

PRECAUTIONS: Very relaxing which is fine, but not if a clear head and concentration is needed.

MIND: Rather hypnotic and somewhat euphoric, said to relieve chronic anxiety, depression and stress. Soothing in highly emotional states, hysteria and shock. Instills a feeling of peace.

BODY: Its tranquillising action on the sympathetic nervous system makes it a good remedy in cases of insomnia, especially where sleep is disturbed due to depression. Also helpful with neuralgia (nerve pain), headaches and vertigo. Said to ease bouts of yawning!

Its calming effect on anxiety could be beneficial to sexual problems and said to be an effective aphrodisiac. Also relieves emotional depression associated with pre menstrual tension and some menopausal symptoms such as irritability and tearfulness.

An antispasmodic action promotes a calming effect on the intestines and can be helpful with colitis and diarrhoea.

Soothes palpitations of the heart and cleanses the blood, improving circulation – generally a very good tonic.

EFFECT ON SKIN: Has pronounced cytophylactic properties, helping with regeneration of skin cells and improving skin elasticity. Dry, sensitive and mature skins seems to benefit most. However, generally helpful with all skin conditions particularly thread veins, scarring and stretch marks. Also said to give some protection to the skin during X-ray treatment.

BLENDS: Benzoin, Bergamot, Coriander, Geranium, Jasmine, Lavender, Lemon, Lime, Orange, Palmarosa, Petitgrain, Rose, Rosemary, Sandalwood, Ylang Ylang.

NIAOULI

Plant/Part	:	Tree/Leaves and Shoots
Latin Name	:	Melaleuca viridiflora
Family	:	Myrtaceae
Note	:	Top
Planet	:	?
Extraction	:	Distillation

AROMA: Slightly sweet, clear and penetrating.

FEATURES: Niaouli is a large tree which grows abundantly in Australia. Its bushy foliage and yellow flowers are also a familiar sight in New Caledonia – a South Sea island where distillation of the oil frequently took place. The healthy air in these regions and the absence of malaria is attributed to this tree. It appears that the falling leaves cover the ground and act like a strong disinfectant.

HISTORY & MYTH: A pronounced effect on bacteria may account for Niaouli's long history of useful service. Effective though it was on many kinds of ailments it was also drunk as a beverage in the Middle East. Sometimes referred to by the French term 'gemenol', though assigned its botanical name in 1788 during Captain Cook's voyage to Australia.

The French found a use for it in their hospital obstetric wards valuing it as a strong antiseptic. It is sometimes used as a substitute for oils of Cajuput and Eucalyptus in the treatment of coughs, rheumatism and neuralgia. A popular ingredient of many pharmaceutical preparations such as toothpastes and mouth sprays.

CHEMICAL CONSTITUENTS: Valeric (Acid), Terpineol (Alcohol), Cineole (Ketone), Limonene, Pinene (Terpenes).

PROPERTIES: Analgesic, Antirheumatic, Antiseptic, Balsamic, Bacteriacide, Cicatrisant, Decongestant, Febrifuge, Insecticide, Stimulant, Vermifuge, Vulnerary.

PRECAUTIONS: ?

MIND: Generally stimulating and reviving, clears the head and may aid concentration.

BODY: A tissue stimulant promoting local circulation, increasing white blood cell and antibody activity, helping to fight infections. A good oil to choose at the beginning of illness to fortify the body and indeed useful in any weakened condition. Though not offering a cure, could be of service in helping to strengthen the immune system with A.I.D.'s patients. Naturally this is best done in co-operation with qualified medical personnel.

Has a decided impact on the respiratory system, dealing with such problems as chest infections, bronchitis, tuberculosis, influenza, pneumonia, whooping cough, asthma, sinusitis, catarrh and laryngitis.

Also has a tonic action on the intestines and may be effective against enteritis, dysentery, intestinal parasites as well as dealing with urinary infections.

Its pain relieving properties seem to give some aid to rheumatism and neuralgia.

EFFECT ON SKIN: Firms the tissues and aids healing and may be helpful with skin eruptions, acne, boils, ulcers, burns and cuts. Useful for washing infected wounds.

BLENDS: Coriander, Fennel, Galbanum, Juniper, Lavender, Lemon, Lime, Myrtle, Orange, Pine, Peppermint, Rosemary.

NUTMEG

Plant/Part	:	Tree/Fruit
Latin Name	:	Myristica fragrans
Family	:	Myristicaceae
Note	:	Top
Planet	:	Jupiter
Extraction	:	Distillation

AROMA: Sharp, spicy, rather musky and warming.

FEATURES: The powerful aroma of Nutmegs perfumes the tropics. They grow on a sturdy evergreen tree which reaches to a height of forty five feet and one male tree is said to pollinate 20 female trees. Though originating from the Molucca Islands the tree is also found in Penang, Java, the West Indies and Sri Lanka. Nutmegs resemble a small peach and tend to vary in size, shape and quality. The oil is obtained from the kernel of the seeds and the husk gives another oil – Mace – which is not easily come by.

HISTORY & MYTH: The use of Nutmeg may be more recent than that of Mace, which was esteemed highly by ancient civilisations. Nutmeg was used for intestinal disorders in India and the Egyptians employed it in embalming. It was an ingredient of Italian incense which guarded against the plague along with Bay, Clove, Juniper, Myrrh, Myrtle and Rose. In the Middle Ages, it became a renowned treatment for piles, grated and mixed with lard to use as an ointment. It was thought to be a stomach strengthener too.

Portugal had monopoly of the spice trade until 1605 when the Dutch took over and ran other vessels out of the water when they came too close to the Moluccas. It was not until 1768 that the Nutmeg, also known as Nux Moschata, was introduced into other countries. Nutmeg has been used in flavouring foods, as an ingredient of liqueurs, dental products, perfumes and many hair lotions.

CHEMICAL CONSTITUENTS: Borneol, Geraniol, Linalool, Terpineol (Alcohols), Eugenol, Myristicin, Safrole (Phenols), Camphene, Dipentene, Pinene (Terpenes).

PROPERTIES: Analgesic, Antispasmodic, Antidontalgic, Antiemetic, Antiseptic, Aphrodisiac, Cardiac, Carminative, Emmenagogue, Laxative, Parturient, Stimulant, Stomachic, Tonic.

PRECAUTIONS: Its best to be cautious with this rather potent oil since prolonged use may over-excite the motor nerves possibly causing mental discomfort. Or at worst delirium and convulsions though conversely may induce numbness. Could also over-stimulate the heart as well as irritate the skin. Best avoided in pregnancy.

MIND: Invigorates and activates the mind and could revive fainting fits.

BODY: Its main action appears to be on the digestive system and particularly useful in breaking down fats and starchy foods as well as encouraging appetite. May have an effect on wind, nausea, chronic vomiting, bad breath and diarrhoea – though apparently averts constipation too. Can act as an intestinal antiseptic and said to dissolve gall stones.

A tonic to the reproductive system since it imitates the hormone oestrogen, regulating scanty periods and soothing pain. Reputedly helpful with sexual problems since it is thought to be an aphrodisiac and not surprisingly, is said to be an aid to birth by strengthening contractions.

Its rather warming quality is a balm to muscular aches and pains as well as rheumatism, especially of the chronic kind. Also said to lesson the sharp stabbing pain associated with neuralgia.

A very stimulating oil invigorating the heart and circulation.

EFFECT ON SKIN: Said to be a good tonic for the hair.

BLENDS: Black Pepper, Cinnamon, Clove, Coriander, Cypress, Frankincense, Galbanum, Lemon, Lime, Melissa, Orange, Patchouli, Rosemary, Ti-Tree.

ORANGE

Plant/Part	:	Fruit/Peel
Latin Name	:	Citrus vulgaris/aurantium/ cinesis
Family	:	Rutaceae
Note	:	Top
Planet	:	Sun
Extraction	:	Expression

AROMA: A zesty and refreshing citrus fragrance.

FEATURES: Three different essential oils from the orange tree spoil us for choice. The cheerful Orange from the peel, Neroli from the lovely white flowers, which hang from the numerous branches, and the intriguing Petitgrain from the leaves. The Orange tree is native to China and India and was brought to Europe around the 17th century. These days it is found abundantly in the Mediterranean region, Israel and the Americas. The essential oil is obtained from both the sweet orange (var. dulcis) and bitter orange (var. amara).

HISTORY & MYTH: Long held to be a symbol of innocence and fertility – opposing qualities one would have thought. However, the Trojan Wars began innocently enough. It was a 'golden apple', said actually to be an Orange, that Paris awarded Venus in a beauty contest. Venus in turn gave Paris the lovely Helen but forgot to mention that the lady was already married. The rest is history.

The Arabic 'Narandj' is the root word for Orange and it is possible that the Crusaders, along with many other spoils, brought the fruit to Europe. Certainly it was known in England around the 16th century. The Orange travelled to California on the boats carrying the early missionaries where an important industry now exists. The peel was used in a West Indian liqueur named Curacao and of course, it also makes a delicious marmalade. The oil is used in perfume and food industries.

CHEMICAL CONSTITUENTS: Nerol (Alcohol), Citral (Aldehyde), Limonene (Terpene), Methyl anthranilate (Ester).

PROPERTIES: Antidepressant, Antiseptic, Antispasmodic, Carminative, Digestive, Febrifuge, Sedative, Stomachic, Tonic.

PRECAUTIONS: Prolonged use and high dosage may irritate sensitive skin and there is a chance of phototoxicity as well.

MIND: Spreads a little sunshine on gloomy thoughts and depression. Dispels tension and stress encouraging a positive outlook. Reviving when feeling bored and lacking in energy.

BODY: Seems to have a very calming action on the stomach especially in nervous states, quells the proverbial butterflies. Physical ailments may be helped too – balancing gastric complaints like diarrhoea and constipation. It also stimulates bile and could help digestion of fats. May well encourage the appetite so beware if dieting.

Aids absorption of vitamin C which action could ward off viral infections. Seems to have a good effect on colds, bronchitis and fever conditions by bringing down temperature.

Helps with the formation of collagen, vital for growth and repair of body tissues and together with its relaxing nature seems to be an effective palliative with painful and sore muscles as well as rickety bones.

Its relaxing nature could be beneficial to insomnia brought on by anxiety. In the same way possibility of bringing down high levels of cholesterol in the blood.

EFFECT ON SKIN: Its sweating action speeds out toxins in a congested skin though at the same time appears to deal effectively with dry skin, wrinkles and dermatitis. All in all a rather good skin tonic.

BLENDS: Angelica, Cinnamon, Coriander, Clove, Cypress, Frankincense, Geranium, Jasmine, Juniper, Lavender, Neroli, Nutmeg, Petitgrain, Rose, Rosewood.

ORIGANUM

Plant/Part	:	Herb/Flowering tops and leaves
Latin Name	:	Origanum vulgare
Family	:	Labiatae
Note	:	Middle
Planet	:	Mercury
Extraction	:	Distillation

AROMA: Herby, woody, yet slightly spicy.

FEATURES: 'Wild Marjoram', as it is otherwise known, originates from the Mediterranean region. Now grown all over Europe as well as the United States and Asia. Its rather hairy and woody stem, bearing ovate leaves and purple/pink flowers, reaches just under three feet. Said to have similar properties to Marjoram (Origanum Marjorana) but is more toxic since it contains 'Thymol'.

HISTORY & MYTH: Origanum was a favourite bath oil with the Egyptians though the Greeks seem to have found a more solemn use for the herb. It was planted in graveyards to help the spirits of the departed achieve peace. Nevertheless it was still used in cooking and medicine – thought to be effective against tuberculosis.

Aristotle is reported to have said that tortoises will eat Origanum after swallowing a snake – which sounds like good news for the tortoise. In Persia, astrologers brewed balms from Origanum as protection against hostile planets! Very few herbs escape being put into love potions and Origanum is no exception. It was however, cultivated in monasteries around the 13th century, but we can probably rest assured that the monks revered it more for its effect on chest complaints than for arousing ardour!

CHEMICAL CONSTITUENTS: Carvacrol, Thymol (Phenols), Cymene, Pinene (Terpenes).

PROPERTIES: Analgesic, Antirheumatic, Antispasmodic, Antiseptic, Aperitif, Bechic, Carminative, Disinfectant, Emmenagogue, Expectorant, Hepatic, Laxative, Parasiticide, Rubefacient, Splenetic, Stimulant, Stomachic, Sudorific, Tonic, Vulnerary.

PRECAUTIONS: A very potent oil and could irritate the mucous membranes. Best avoided in pregnancy and some say altogether.

MIND: Could be a tonic and stimulant to the nerves though Valnet talks about it being helpful for imaginary or mental diseases – not to mention psychopaths!

BODY: The main effect seems to be on the digestive system, soothing the stomach, liver and spleen. Though probably a tonic and general cleanser as well since it acts on nervous stomach disorders and calms intestinal spasm. May also combat acidity, wind and encourage appetite. Said to be beneficial to aerophagia (swallowing gulps of air).

Appears to have a beneficial action on the respiratory system – colds, bronchitis, catarrh may be relieved. Possibly alleviates symptoms of asthma and whooping cough.

Its stimulating action revives the senses, indeed Culpeper maintains that it could ease deafness, pain and noise in the ears as well as toothache. Seems to have some effect with migraine and facial tics.

Its warming and pain relieving action may be beneficial to period cramps, rheumatism and muscular pain generally. Gives a feeling of well-being.

Reputedly deals with water-logged tissues through its sweating action and possibly encourages flow of urine.

EFFECT ON SKIN: Infected cuts and wounds may respond favourably and apparently has some effect on pediculosis (infestation by skin parasites).

BLENDS: Angelica, Basil, Fennel, Geranium, Lemongrass, Myrtle, Pine, Thyme, Rosemary.

PALMAROSA

Plant/Part	:	Grass/Leaves
Latin Name	:	Cymbopogon martini
Family	:	Gramineae
Note	:	Top
Planet	:	?
Extraction	:	Distillation

AROMA: Sweet, floral slightly dry with a hint of rose.

FEATURES: Distilled from a spreading wild grass which is harvested before the flowers appear. The highest yield of oil is obtained when the grass is fully dried – about one week after it has been cut. Originally from India where the oil has been distilled for generations by highly skilled craftsmen. Also obtained from the Comora Islands and Madagascar. The grass occurs in two varieties, motia and sofia, which grow in different environments and altitudes, the former yielding the better quality oil and finer aroma.

HISTORY & MYTH: Also known as 'Indian Geranium Oil' as well as 'Rosha' and often used to adulterate the more expensive Rose. Oil from sofia is sometimes referred to as 'Gingergrass' which has a lower percentage of geraniol. Occasionally it is mixed with the finer motia though native dealers evaluate good quality oil by hitting the bottle against the palm of the hand. If the air bubbles rising to the surface disappear quickly, the oil is assumed to be normal. Exporters in Bombay assess Palmarosa oil by a simple solubility test.

Palmarosa has also been harvested in the Seychelles producing a softer odour and Java which has a more fruity note. Much of the oil is generally exported to Europe, America and Japan. An ingredient of soaps, cosmetics and perfumes as well as flavouring tobacco.

CHEMICAL CONSTITUENTS: Geraniol, Citronellol, Farnesol (Alcohols), Citral, Citronellal (Aldehydes), Geranyl acetate (Ester), Dipentene, Limonene (Terpenes).

PROPERTIES: Antiseptic, Antiviral, Bacteriacide, Cytophylactic, Febrifuge.

PRECAUTIONS: ?

MIND: Has a calming yet uplifting effect on the emotions. Also said to be able to refresh and clarify the mind.

BODY: Seems to be helpful when the body is overheated and possibly effective in cases of fever by reducing temperature. This enhances its antiviral action since bacteria is weakened in a cool environment.

Acts as a tonic to the digestive system and said to have a beneficial effect on pathogens in the intestinal flora. Could therefore be useful in dysentery and it also has a strengthening effect on stomach muscles. Stimulates the appetite and may be helpful to people suffering from anorexia nervosa since it appears to have such a positive influence on the feelings.

According to Guenther's 'Essential Oils', Gingergrass oil is said to ease stiff joints, possibly its cousin, Palmarosa, might have the same effect.

EFFECT ON SKIN: Restores water balance and stimulates natural secretion of sebum which sounds like a useful oil for dry skin. It also helps skin regrowth by aiding cell regeneration. Though its reputation for eradicating wrinkles must be put to the test! Said to help with general skin infections.

BLENDS: Bergamot, Citronella, Geranium, Jasmine, Lavender, Lime, Melissa, Orange, Petitgrain, Rose, Rosewood, Sandalwood, Violet, Ylang Ylang.

PARSLEY

Plant/Part	:	Herb/Seed
Latin Name	:	Petroselinum sativum
Family	:	Umbelliferae
Note	:	Middle
Planet	:	Mercury
Extraction	:	Distillation

AROMA: Somewhat herby with spicy undertones.

FEATURES: The Greek 'Petros', which gives Parsley its name, means stone and its that kind of gravelly environment that Parsley favours. Originally from the Mediterranean region it now grows abundantly in most continents. There are many varieties of Parsley with either flat or frilled bright green leaves and yellow flowers – the stems reaching to about two feet. France seems to produce a great deal of the essential oil.

HISTORY & MYTH: The practical Egyptians saw Parsley as a remedy for urinary problems whereas the Greeks thought it a symbol of fame and joy. Victors at the Isthmian Games were often crowned with Parsley garlands though it was also included in funeral banquets.

The Romans doubted its merits and firmly believed that it would cause sterility. Indeed they also warned expectant mothers to stay clear of it in case of epilepsy occurring in the infant. Legend associates it with witchcraft bringing 'bad luck' if transplanted. Yet it was very popular in Europe around the 16th century good sense having prevailed. Perhaps the people knew that Parsley is full of vitamins especially iron and vitamin C.

CHEMICAL CONSTITUENTS: Apiol, Myristicin (Phenols), Pinene (Terpene).

PROPERTIES: Antiseptic, Antispasmodic, Aphrodisiac, Carminative, Depurative, Digestive, Diuretic, Expectorant, Emmenagogue, Febrifuge, Laxative, Parturient, Sedative, Tonic.

PRECAUTIONS: A few warnings to be taken into account with this powerful oil. Care is needed with dosage otherwise dizziness may result. Should not be used in pregnancy nor during painful menstruation as it may induce contractions of the womb. Said to have a stimulating and tonic effect on the kidneys, but best avoided in cases of kidney disease and peptic ulcers. Debatable whether should be used in massage.

MIND: An overburdened mind and jangling nerves might benefit from its general cleansing and cooling action.

BODY: A very strong diuretic often helpful in cases of water retention during menstruation as well as in cases of oedema and cellulite. It stimulates the kidneys and could effectively clear cystitis and urinary stones.

Well known for dealing with scanty menstruation as it imitates the oestrogen hormone which could also assuage some menopausal problems. It seems a rather useful oil in childbirth since it stimulates contractions during labour and restores the regenerative system thereafter. Could well promote flow of breast milk and seems to relieve hardening of the breasts.

It has a cleansing action on the blood and a tonic effect on the circulation which may well help to ease rheumatism and arthritis. May also reduce muscle spasm and said to relieve sprains.

Whilst having a calming action on the digestion, it also stimulates the appetite. Useful too with flatulence, comforting any feelings of nausea and cramp and deals with chills of the stomach. May be helpful with piles and acts as a tonic to the liver.

Takes the sting out of insect bites apparently.

EFFECT ON SKIN: Clears wounds and bruises by stimulating the blood flow. Also said to be a tonic to the scalp and hair – and the merest mention of Parsley seems to keep head lice away.

BLENDS: Lavender, Lime, Mandarin, Marjoram, Orange, Rosemary.

PATCHOULI

Plant/Part	:	Shrub/Leaves
Latin Name	:	Pogostemon patchouli
Family	:	Labiatae
Note	:	Base
Planet	:	Sun
Extraction	:	Distillation

AROMA: A strong, earthy and exotic fragrance yet sweet and spicy too.

FEATURES: A bush plant with furry leaves, four inches long and five inches across. The white flowers have a purple hue and the plant itself grows to about three feet. Its a soil exhausting shrub and needs fertile ground to thrive. The oil is obtained from the young leaves which are dried and fermented prior to distillation. The oil, like a good wine, improves with age and gives a fuller odour. Produced in India, Malaysia, Burma, Paraguay.

HISTORY & MYTH: The name 'Patchouli' is from the Hindustan and has a long history of medicinal use in Malaysia, China, India and Japan. It was a renowned antidote against insect and snake bite. The greater volume of oil was distilled in British Malaya for many years but the Seychelles became large producers during the last World War – though the oil is said to be slightly inferior to the Malay.

Dried patchouli leaves were placed amongst the folds of Indian cashmere shawls in Victorian times to protect the merchandise from moths. In India, Patchouli sachets are a popular way to perfume linen and keep an eye on bedbugs. A base fixative of oriental type perfumes, it was much in vogue during the 'Flower Power' era of the 1960's along with Sandalwood and Jasmine.

CHEMICAL CONSTITUENTS: Patchoulol (Alcohol), Benzoic, Cinnamic (Aldehydes), Eugenol (Phenol), Cadinene (Sesquiterpene).

PROPERTIES: Antidepressant, Antiphlogistic, Antiseptic, Aphrodisiac, Astringent, Cicatrisant, Cytophylactic, Deodorant, Diuretic, Febrifuge, Fungicide, Insecticide, Sedative, Tonic.

PRECAUTIONS: Apparently sedative in low doses and rather stimulating in high. May cause loss of appetite which is fine if eating habits need to be curbed. Also, its odour may be a little persistent for some people.

MIND: Its rather earthy aura promotes a grounding and balancing effect. Seems to banish lethargy and sharpen the wits, thereby clarifying problems and making the mind more objective.

BODY: Perhaps Patchouli's most outstanding feature is its binding action due to strong astringent and cicatrisant properties. This could be helpful for loose skin especially after excessive dieting. Since it also seems to curb appetite its probably useful for overall weight reduction. Could well be helpful in cases of diarrhoea too.

Seems to have marked diuretic properties which could prove valuable in cases of water retention and cellulite. Also said to offset heavy sweating, though certainly has a marked deodorising action, helpful when feeling hot and bothered.

There is some association between Patchouli and increasing libido. Its bracing action on the central nervous system may account for this! However, it is neither too sedative nor too stimulating which effectively assists feelings of balance.

In any event, it seems to relieve the nasty effects from insect and snake bites!

EFFECT ON SKIN: Said to be a tissue regenerator helping regrowth of skin cells and forming scar tissue. Apparently cools inflamed conditions and heals rough, cracked skin, sores and wounds. Some relief may also be obtained from acne, eczema, fungal infections and scalp disorders.

BLENDS: Bergamot, Black Pepper, Clary Sage, Elemi, Frankincense, Galbanum, Geranium, Ginger, Lavender, Lemongrass, Myrrh, Neroli, Pine, Rose, Rosewood, Sandalwood.

PEPPERMINT

Plant/Part	:	Herb/Leaves and Flowering tops
Latin Name	:	Mentha piperita
Family	:	Labiatae
Note	:	Top
Planet	:	Venus or Mercury
Extraction	:	Distillation

AROMA: Strongly piercing, sharp, menthol fragrance.

FEATURES: This herb of many species is a native of Europe but also grows in Japan as well as the USA, now the main producer of Peppermint. Apparently the best type is from England since the plant favours the damp conditions – even if no-one else does! The stem reaches to about three feet and has slightly hairy serrated leaves with purple spiked flowers. It is a hybrid of Watermint (M. Aquatica) and Spearmint (M. Spicata).

HISTORY & MYTH: Like many other herbs it was known to the ancient Egyptians, Greeks and Romans. The latter crowned themselves with Peppermint at their feasts, aware of its detoxifying effects no doubt! However, they were not averse to using it as an ingredient of wine.

It was a perfume component amongst the Hebrews reputedly because of its aphrodisiac properties. They may have heard about the nymph Mentha who was hotly pursued by Pluto. Persephone, his jealous wife then hounded the poor girl and trod her ferociously into the ground. Pluto, with rare compassion, changed Mentha into a herb. Notwithstanding all this, it has been cultivated commercially in England since 1750.

CHEMICAL CONSTITUENTS: Menthol (Alcohol), Menthyl acetate (Ester), Carvone, Jasmone, Menthone (Ketones), Carvacrol (Phenol), Limonene, Phellandrene (Terpenes).

PROPERTIES: Analgesic, Antidontalgic, Anaesthetic, Antigalactagogue, Antiphlogistic, Antiseptic, Antispasmodic, Astringent, Carminative, Cephalic, Cholagogue, Cordial, Decongestant, Emmenagogue, Expectorant, Febrifuge, Hepatic, Nervine, Stimulant, Stomachic, Sudorific, Vasoconstrictor, Vermifuge.

PRECAUTIONS: A powerful and overwhelming aroma so care should be taken with dosage. Probably best use is in infusers rather than massage though might be okay in local areas. It is likely to irritate the skin and mucous membranes however, and certainly should be kept well away from the eyes. Best avoided in pregnancy and by nursing mothers since could discourage flow of milk. May antidote homeopathic remedies.

MIND: Its cooling nature seems to relieve states of anger, hysteria and nervous trembling. Excellent for mental fatigue and depression.

BODY: Has a dual action – cooling when hot and warming when cold. This makes it a good remedy for colds by halting mucous and fevers and encouraging perspiration. Useful in respiratory disorders generally as well as dry coughs and sinus congestion. Reputedly has an effect on asthma, bronchitis, cholera, pneumonia and tuberculosis.

Its action on the digestive system of paramount importance, particularly in acute conditions. Has a relaxing and slightly anaesthetic effect on stomach muscles. Apparently beneficial against food poisoning and deals with vomiting, diarrhoea and constipation, flatulence, halitosis, colic, gall stones and nausea as well as travel sickness. May be helpful for kidney and liver disorders.

Stimulating qualities valuable for general numbness of the limbs, as well as shock, vertigo, anaemia, dizziness and fainting – producing a tonic to the heart and mind. Its cooling and pain relieving action seems to ease headaches, migraines and toothache. It is an excellent remedy for aching feet and some relief may also be gained from rheumatism, neuralgia and muscular aches.

Scanty menstruation, painful periods and mastitis could well respond to this useful oil.

However, not much liked by insects and vermin!

EFFECT ON SKIN: By removing toxic congestion, could help cases of dermatitis, ringworm, scabies and pruritus. Due to capillary constriction, it is cooling in action and can relieve itching, inflammation and sunburn. Also softens skin, helps to remove blackheads and effective on greasy skin and hair.

BLENDS: Benzoin, Cedarwood, Cypress, Lavender, Mandarin, Marjoram, Niaouli, Pine, Rosemary.

PETITGRAIN

Plant/Part	:	Orange Tree/Leaves and young shoots
Latin Name	:	Citrus vulgaris/aurantium
Family	:	Rutaceae
Note	:	Middle to Top
Planet	:	Sun
Extraction	:	Distillation

AROMA: A rather haunting fragrance alternately woody and floral.

FEATURES: One of the three oils obtained from the Orange tree, the others being Neroli from the flowers and Orange from the fruit. A native of central Asia, now found mainly in the Mediterranean region with essential oil produced by Italy, Spain and Paraguay. The best oil however, is said to come from France, though the high price once led to adulteration using a mixture of the bitter and sweet oranges.

HISTORY & MYTH: The name means 'little grains' as Petitgrain was originally distilled from the unripe fruit rather than the leaves. Other sources of this oil come from Lemon and Mandarin trees. Once the leaves were used to treat epilepsy. These days, however, the distilled oil is widely employed in pharmaceuticals and perfumery, indeed it is a popular ingredient of many colognes.

CHEMICAL CONSTITUENTS: Geraniol, Linalool, Nerol, Terpineol (Alcohol), Citral (Aldehyde), Geranyl Acetate, Linalyl Acetate (Ester), Camphene, Limonene (Terpenes).

PROPERTIES: Antidepressant, Antispasmodic, Deodorant, Sedative.

PRECAUTIONS: ?

MIND: Calms anger and panic, gives assurance when feeling down and refreshes the mind. A soothing action on the emotions parallels the effect of Neroli though the latter oil may deal more effectively with serious states of depression.

BODY: A sedative of the nervous system, its relaxing properties an aid to anxiety when accompanied by rapid heart beat or insomnia. Seems to slow the body down, eases breathing and relaxes muscle spasm.

Helpful in debilitated states after illness since it seems to act as a mild immuno-stimulant, encouraging general resistance to illness. At the same time, its deodorising properties could help refresh and revive the body.

Reputedly helpful with painful digestion by calming stomach muscles.

EFFECT ON SKIN: A tonic effect on the skin could help in clearing up skin blemishes like pimples or even acne.

BLENDS: Bergamot, Cedarwood, Cardamom, Geranium, Lavender, Melissa, Neroli, Orange, Palmarosa, Rosemary, Rosewood, Sandalwood, Ylang Ylang.

PIMENTO

Plant/Part	:	Tree/Leaf/Fruit
Latin Name	:	Pimenta officinalis
Family	:	Myrtaceae
Note	:	Top
Planet	:	?
Extraction	:	Distillation

AROMA: Warm, spicy and pungent.

FEATURES: Pimento is found all over the West Indies – its original home – though it can also be traced to South America, Reunion and India. An evergreen tree reaching to about thirty feet it has small white flowers and green fruits which change to a reddish brown. The plant is distilled in water where it separates into two portions, a lighter fraction floating on top and a heavier one sinking to the bottom. The two are mixed to obtain the usual oil.

HISTORY & MYTH: Also known as 'Allspice' probably because its flavour resembles a mixture of Pepper, Clove and Cinnamon. It is one of the main exports from Jamaica and sometimes referred to as 'Jamaica Pepper' as well. The leaf oil – distillation began in 1916 – was a late starter compared to the berry oil.

The Aztecs used it in a beverage called 'Chocolada' and these days appears in a popular West Indian drink called 'Pimento Dram' as well as being an ingredient of Bay Rum. Portuguese traders introduced Pimento to Europe and it is now frequently used in Northern Europe usually as a condiment and in flavouring food.

CHEMICAL CONSTITUENTS: Cineole (Ketone), Eugenol (Phenol), Caryophyllene (Sesquiterpene), Phellandrene (Terpene).

PROPERTIES: Analgesic, Antidontalgic, Antidepressant, Aphrodisiac, Carminative, Rubefacient, Stomachic, Tonic.

PRECAUTIONS: Careful over dosage as may irritate the skin and mucous membranes. Debatable whether should be used in massage since it is such a powerful oil though might be fine in local areas.

MIND: Warming to the emotions when feeling cold and dejected. Gives a boost to the mind in states of tiredness and exhaustion.

BODY: A very warming oil – gets the circulation going – and helpful in conditions of extreme cold. Often beneficial for coughs and chest infections as well as influenza, colds and bronchitis.

Soothing to the gastro-intestinal tract, especially for gripping pains leading to stomach ache, flatulence, intestinal pain and vomiting. May also have an effect on diarrhoea.

Its analgesic properties seem to ease cramps and muscle pain as in rheumatism and arthritis. Could relieve headaches and toothache.

A good overall tonic to the body.

EFFECT ON SKIN: ?

BLENDS: Frankincense, Galbanum, Ginger, Lavender, Lemon, Lemongrass, Nutmeg, Orange, Pine.

PINE

Plant/Part	:	Tree/Needles and cones
Latin Name	:	Pinus sylvestris
Family	:	Pinaceae
Note	:	Middle
Planet	:	Mars
Extraction	:	Distillation

AROMA: A fresh forest fragrance.

FEATURES: A large conifer, found mainly in Northern Europe, North East Russia and Scandinavia. There are about 80 species of this magnificent tree and much of the oil is obtained mainly from the Scots and Norwegian Pine. Generally has a reddish bark with needle-like grey-green leaves and orange-yellow flowers.

HISTORY & MYTH: Hardly a stranger to the ancient civilisations of Egypt, Greece and Arabia who recognised its strong curative properties. Though it has some association with religious ceremonies, it was particularly useful in pulmonary infections like bronchitis, tuberculosis and pneumonia. Inhalations were the primary method of use. Indeed, it is said that people flock to areas of abundant pine growth since the air there is excellent for lung complaints.

The North American Indians however, thought it did a good job with scurvy. A very familiar ingredient of soaps and bath salts, valuable for its deodorising and disinfectant properties.

CHEMICAL CONSTITUENTS: Borneol (Alcohol), Bornyl acetate, Terpinyl acetate (Esters), Cadinene (Sesquiterpene), Camphene, Dipentene, Phellandrene, Pinene, Sylvestrene (Terpenes).

PROPERTIES: Antiphlogistic, Antiseptic, Balsamic, Decongestant, Deodorant, Diuretic, Disinfectant, Expectorant, Restorative, Rubefacient, Sudorific, Stimulant, Tonic.

PRECAUTIONS: Dwarf Pine (Pinus Pumilio), another more toxic species, should be avoided. Our P. Sylvestris is fine in small doses though it may irritate sensitive skins.

MIND: Good for feelings of weakness, general debility and mental fatigue. Gives a refreshing note to a tired mind.

BODY: A powerful antiseptic and helpful in cases of bronchitis, laryngitis and influenza. It is both warming and cooling depending upon the body's needs. Generally has a good effect on respiratory problems, eases breathlessness and helps to clear the sinuses. Seems to have some effect on profuse sweating.

A general kidney cleanser and known to be effective with cystitis, hepatitis and prostate problems. Reduces inflammation of the gall-bladder and puts a ban on gall-stones. Said to stimulate the adrenal glands producing a revitalising effect on the body.

It also stimulates the circulation and with its warming properties may relieve rheumatism, gout, sciatica and arthritis – often used in compresses when these conditions are very painful. Could be beneficial for muscular pain and stiffness generally,

Seems to give some relief to digestive problems particularly intestinal disturbances.

Also said to stem leucorrhoea in women and may have some effect on metritis (inflammation of the uterus). Reputedly effective on male sexual problems, possibly impotence.

Fleas, it is said, just cannot abide the odour of Pine!

EFFECT ON SKIN: Valuable for congested skins and said to have some effect with eczema and psoriasis. Seems to have a healing action on cuts and skin irritations.

BLENDS: Cedarwood, Cinnamon, Clove, Cypress, Eucalyptus, Lavender, Myrtle, Niaouli, Rosemary, Thyme, Ti-Tree.

ROSE

Plant/Part	:	Flower/Petals
Latin Lane	:	Rosa centifolia (Cabbage Rose) Rosa damascena (Damask Rose) Rosa gallica (Red Rose)
Family	:	Rosaceae
Note	:	Middle to Base
Planet	:	Venus
Extraction	:	Enfleurage

AROMA: Deep, sweet and flowery – an exquisite perfume.

FEATURES: A favourite flower of many countries though the oil is mainly obtained from Morocco, Turkey and France. Damask Rose, also known as Rose Otto, comes from Bulgaria. Cultivated in mountainous regions, it has to be picked just after the dew and distilled immediately to maximise on oil yield. The enfleurage method of extraction yields greater quantities of oil and is known as absolute.

HISTORY & MYTH: Rose was possibly the first plant used in distillation credited to Avicenna, the 10th century Arab physician. A very popular plant in the East, Persian warriors adorned their shields with red roses and the conquering Turks introduced it to Bulgaria in 17th century.

Long a symbol of love and purity – the petals were scattered at weddings to ensure a happy marriage. Rose was probably an aid to meditation and prayer since the story goes that St Dominic (1170–1221) was visited by the Virgin Mary in a mystical vision and received the first rosary – each bead was scented with roses. The Buddhists and Moslems also use a form of rosary.

Rosa Gallica, known as the 'Apothecary's Rose', was used in healing balms for lung diseases and asthma in the Middle Ages. When scented food became the rage in Elizabethan times the aroma of Rose was a favourite. During the last World War vitamin C was in short supply and Rosehips were used instead. The previous century saw a rapid rise in the French Rose industry and the oil remains a popular ingredient in perfumes and soaps.

CHEMICAL CONSTITUENTS: Geranic (Acid), Citronnellol, Geraniol, Farnesol, Nerol (Alcohols), Eugenol (Phenol), Myrcene (Terpene).

PROPERTIES: Antidepressant, Antiphlogistic, Antiseptic, Antispasmodic, Aphrodisiac, Bacteriacide, Cholagogue, Depurative, Diuretic, Emmenagogue, Haemostatic, Hepatic, Laxative, Sedative, Splenetic, Stomachic, Tonic.

PRECAUTIONS: Since it is an emmenagogue best avoided in pregnancy.

MIND: Has a soothing effect on the emotions, particularly depression, grief, jealousy and resentment. Lifts the heart and eases nervous tension and stress. Its an ultra feminine oil apparently – gives a woman positive feelings about herself.

BODY: An excellent tonic for the womb, calming pre menstrual tension, promoting vaginal secretions and regulating the menstrual cycle. Its beneficial action on infertility aids 'male' problems too probably by increasing the semen. Helpful with sexual difficulties, particularly frigidity and impotence, soothing the underlying tension and stress by releasing the 'happy' hormone dopamine.

Seems to have a tonic action on the heart by activating sluggish blood circulation, relieving cardiac congestion and toning the capillaries.

Balances and strengthens the stomach during emotional upsets and through its antiseptic and purging action, helps to clear the alimentary canal. To some extent relieves nausea, vomiting and constipation.

The ancient Romans valued it for hangovers possibly because of its cleansing and purging action on toxins – alcoholic excess would of course congest the liver. Possibly helps with cases of jaundice.

Apparently has a soothing action on sore throats and eases coughs.

EFFECT ON SKIN: Useful for all skin types though particularly good for mature, dry, hard or sensitive skin. Its tonic and soothing quality is helpful for inflammation and a constricting action on the capillaries is a valuable treatment for broken thread veins.

BLENDS: Bergamot, Chamomile, Clary Sage, Galbanum, Geranium, Jasmine, Lavender, Neroli, Orange, Palmarosa, Patchouli, Sandalwood.

ROSEMARY

Plant/Part	:	Herb/Flowering tops and leaves
Latin Name	:	Rosmarinus officinalis
Family	:	Labiatae
Note	:	Middle
Planet	:	Sun
Extraction	:	Distillation

AROMA: Strong, clear and penetrating, a refreshing herbal fragrance.

FEATURES: Rosemary takes its name from the Latin Rosmarinus or sea dew as it is rather fond of water. The woody stem which grows to about three feet supports dark green linear leaves and bees go wild for the bluish/lilac flowers. Originally from Asia, Rosemary has become a familiar sight in the Mediterranean region and much of the essential oil is obtained from France, Tunisia and Yugoslavia.

HISTORY & MYTH: Traces of Rosemary have been found in Egyptian tombs and indeed the Greeks and Romans saw it as a symbol of regeneration as well. They held it to be a sacred plant, giving comfort to the living and peace to the dead. Rosemary sprigs adorned their gods and it was used as incense to drive away evil spirits. The Moors however, thought it would ward off pests and planted Rosemary bushes in their orchards.

Its rejuvenating properties seem to have worked for Donna Isabella, the Queen of Hungary, who in her advanced years used it as a face wash. Apparently it restored her youthful looks! Since Rosemary has always been used to preserve meat there might be some substance in this miracle. Other ingredients were supposedly Lemon, Rose, Neroli, Melissa and Peppermint. Its antiseptic properties were also recognised in French hospitals where it was burnt during epidemics.

CHEMICAL CONSTITUENTS: Borneol (Alcohol), Cuminic (Aldehyde), Bornyl acetate (Ester), Camphor, Cineole (Ketones), Caryophyllene (Sesquiterpene), Camphene, Pinene (Terpenes).

PROPERTIES: Analgesic, Antidepressant, Antirheumatic, Antiseptic, Antispasmodic, Astringent, Carminative, Cephalic, Cholagogue, Cicatrisant, Cordial, Digestive, Diuretic, Emmenagogue, Hepatic, Hypertensive, Nervine, Resolvent, Stimulant, Stomachic, Sudorific, Tonic, Vulnerary.

PRECAUTIONS: Its highly stimulating action may not be suitable for people with epilepsy or high blood pressure. Best avoided in pregnancy too since it is an emmenagogue. Might antidote homeopathic remedies.

MIND: Enlivens the brain cells, clears the head and aids memory. Good for mental strain, general dullness and lethargy. It is very invigorating and strengthens the mind when there is weakness and exhaustion.

BODY: Energises and activates the brain, the vital part of the central nervous system. Seems to revive the senses and in some cases could play a part in restoring impediments of speech, hearing and sight. Clears headaches and migraines especially when connected to gastric problems. May be helpful for vertigo. A good nerve stimulant and helps to tone temporarily paralysed limbs.

A pain relieving agent without being too sedative, helps ease gout, rheumatic pains and tired over-worked muscles.

A valuable heart tonic and cardiac stimulant, normalising low blood pressure. Possibly good effect on anaemia. A tonic for the lungs and could help with colds, asthma, chronic bronchitis and influenza.

Acts as a liver decongestant and may help to relieve hepatitis and cirrhosis as well as gall stones, jaundice or bile duct blockage. A boosting action on the digestion could ease colitis, dyspepsia, flatulence and stomach pains.

Seems to relieve menstrual cramp and combats scanty periods. Its diuretic properties useful with water retention during menstruation and may be effective with cellulite and obesity.

EFFECT ON SKIN: Helpful for sagging skin as Rosemary is a strong astringent – toning and binding – and may ease congestion, puffiness and swellings as well. Its stimulating action found to benefit scalp disorders and could alleviate dandruff and encourage hair growth.

BLENDS: Basil, Cedarwood, Frankincense, Geranium, Ginger, Grapefruit, Lemongrass, Lime, Mandarin, Melissa, Myrtle, Orange, Peppermint, Tangerine.

ROSEWOOD

Plant/Part	:	Tree/Wood
Latin Name	:	Aniba rosaeaodora
Family	:	Lauraceae
Note	:	Top to Middle
Planet	:	Sun?
Extraction	:	Distillation

AROMA: Sweet, woody, floral and slightly spicy.

FEATURES: This beautiful oil is distilled from the heartwood of an evergreen tree found in the tropical rain forests of Brazil. It grows to almost one hundred and twenty five feet and has yellow flowers. Prior to 1927, the oil was largely obtained from French Guiana where it was called 'Cayenne' oil, after the capital city. The two oils are distilled from trees belonging to closely related species. The heavy wood resembles mahogany, though the Brazilian is a more grey yellow colour. Prior to distillation the wood is reduced to chips and the Cayenne variety echoes Lily of the Valley.

HISTORY & MYTH: 'Bois de Rose' is a kind of nom de plume some suppliers use although its known locally in Brazil as 'Jacaranda'. Long established in perfumery – probably under another variety Convulvus scoparious – Rosewood has only recently been introduced into Aromatherapy. The rose scented heartwood was often used to make cabinets in France as well as brush and knife handles.

The trees were shipped to Europe from French Guiana for distilling but soaring freight rates saw the rise of distilleries locally. A huge demand meant that other sources were sought and eventually found in Brazil where the tree grows profusely in the wild. The Brazilian essential oil output is vast and to prevent extinction of trees, the government has enacted legislation requiring distilleries to plant a new tree for each one cut down.

CHEMICAL CONSTITUENTS: Geraniol, Linalool, Nerol, Terpineol (Alcohol), Cineole (Ketone), Dipentene (Terpene).

PROPERTIES: Analgesic, Antidepressant, Antiseptic, Aphrodisiac, Bacteriacide, Cephalic, Deodorant, Insecticide, Stimulant, Tonic.

PRECAUTIONS: ?

MIND: Said to stabilize the Central Nervous System and could therefore have an overall balancing effect. Seems to be helpful when feeling low, weary and over-burdened with problems – gives an uplifting, enlivening effect.

BODY: A first rate remedy for chronic complaints it seems, particularly where the immune system has been under par, giving it a helpful boost. Possibly effective in fighting micro-organisms and viruses and valuable as an antiseptic for the throat. A palliative for ticklish coughs.

Acclaimed aphrodisiac properties may work wonders in restoring libido and could have some effect on sexual problems such as impotence and frigidity. Reputedly helpful for people who have suffered sexual abuse and its comforting and warming action may rekindle dormant sensual feelings.

Its cephalic quality may relieve headaches especially when accompanied by nausea – probably mitigates some of the effects of jet-lag too.

A positive deodorising action helps the body cope with excess heat and moisture. Seems to be valuable as an insect repellent.

EFFECT ON SKIN: Apparently a cell stimulant and tissue regenerator which action could be useful with cuts and wounds. Reputedly helpful with skin that is dry, sensitive and inflamed. May even combat ageing skin and wrinkles! Its balancing and warming action possibly valuable for hydrated conditions as well.

BLENDS: Cedarwood, Coriander, Frankincense, Geranium, Palmarosa, Patchouli, Petitgrain, Rose, Rosemary, Sandalwood, Vetivert.

SAGE

Plant/Part	:	Herb/Leaves and flowers
Latin Name	:	Salvia officinalis
Family	:	Labiatae
Note	:	Top
Planet	:	Jupiter
Extraction	:	Distillation

AROMA: Clear, herbal and sharp.

FEATURES: Sage usually has purple green leaves and blue flowers though indeed, there are many varieties of this attractive plant. It tends to reach to about two feet and grows wild in Yugoslavia and Dalmatia. Said to originate from the Mediterranean region from where a great deal of the oil is obtained.

HISTORY & MYTH: The Chinese were keen on Sage believing it cured sterility. The Romans thought it would heal just about anything. They saw it as a miracle plant and indeed, the root word from the Latin 'salvare' means 'to heal' or to 'save'. With its association with wisdom and ability to bestow 'long life', it remained a very popular herb throughout the centuries.

It was an ingredient of many nerve tonics during the Middle Ages and the actual herb was used to clean gums and whiten teeth. Sage tea was a popular beverage in England before China and India tea were imported. The essential oil tends to be used in masculine perfumes.

CHEMICAL CONSTITUENTS: Borneol, Salviol (Alcohol), Camphor, Cineole, Thujone (Ketones), Phellandrene (Terpenes).

PROPERTIES: Antigalactagogue, Antirheumatic, Antispasmodic, Antiseptic, Antisudorific, Aperitif, Astringent, Cicatrisant, Depurative, Diuretic, Emmenagogue, Hepatic, Hypertensive, Tonic.

PRECAUTIONS: A powerful oil and in extreme cases may adversely affect the central nervous system by either producing convulsions, epileptic fits or paralysis. Even in low dosage can be toxic. Should not be used in pregnancy nor during breast feeding as it can stem the flow of milk. May also induce excessive uterine spasm. Clary Sage (Salvia Sclarea) has similar curative properties and is thought to be a safer alternative.

MIND: In very small doses, can have a calming effect on the nerves by soothing the parasympathetic nervous system. Indicated for tiredness, depression and grief. Quickens the senses and aids memory apparently.

BODY: Has a beneficial effect on the female reproductive system since it imitates the hormone oestrogen, thereby regulating the menstrual cycle. Retains a good reputation for its effect on sterility and could aid conception. Also valuable for menopausal problems, particularly excessive sweating. Said to treat vaginal thrush.

A tonic for the digestive system and indicated where there is loss of appetite. A very good digestive especially if lots of meat is eaten and a relief for constipation. Helps with the flow of urine and may be a tonic to the liver and kidneys. Effective against water retention and cases of oedema.

Clears mucous from the palate, throat and stomach it seems and possibly has a healing action on mouth ulcers and gingivitis.

May also have an effect on glandular disorders by helping lymphatic flow. Apparently raises low blood pressure as it has a cleansing action on the circulatory system.

Could also be helpful with colds, catarrh, bronchitis and bacterial infections generally. Controls perspiration especially when combined with Bay apparently – though this really would be a potent duo!

Its pain relieving action can be helpful with over-exercised or limp muscles. Useful in cases of fibrositis (a kind of inflammation of muscle) and torticollis (general stiff neck). Eases trembling and palsy.

EFFECT ON SKIN: Seems to arrest bleeding from cuts and wounds and helps the formation of scar tissue. Could also be effective on large pores. Skin problems such as sores, dermatitis, psoriasis and ulcers may also be eased. The herb puts a shine on dull hair – maybe the oil can do the same.

BLENDS: Bay, Bergamot, Geranium, Ginger, Lavender, Melissa, Myrtle, Niaouli, Orange, Rosemary.

SANDALWOOD

Plant/Part	:	Tree/Inner heartwood
Latin Name	:	Santalum album
Family	:	Santalaceae
Note	:	Base
Planet	:	?
Extraction	:	Distillation

AROMA: Woody, sweet and exotic, subtle and lingering.

FEATURES: This beautiful oil comes from a parasitic, evergreen tree which burrows its roots into other trees. The yellowish wood is sold in thin scrapings and the trees are cut when they reach maturity at sixty years – never before thirty. Its commonly agreed that the best essential oil comes from Mysore In india. There are other varieties of Sandalwood such as the red 'Pterocarpus santalinus', used mainly as a colouring agent and the Australian Sandalwood, known as 'Santalum Spicatum', said to produce an inferior oil.

HISTORY & MYTH: Popular since antiquity and caravans loaded with Sandalwood were a familiar sight along the trade routes from India to Egypt, Greece and Rome. Many old Indian temples, as well as furniture, were built from Sandalwood probably because of its resistance to ants. Much in demand as incense – its calming effect was a useful aid to meditation and its popularity in religious ceremonies, especially in India and China, has hardly waned. It was burnt at funerals, reputedly to help free the soul in death.

Used in embalming by the Egyptians it was also a well know remedy in the treatment of gonorrhoea. A frequently used ingredient of perfumes though unfortunately, said to be subject to adulteration. The trees are nearly extinct and now only used for distillation of oil.

CHEMICAL CONSTITUENTS: Santalol (Alcohol), Furfurol (Aldehyde), Santalene (Sesquiterpene).

PROPERTIES: Antiphlogistic, Antiseptic, Antispasmodic, Aphrodisiac, Astringent, Bechic, Carminative, Diuretic, Emollient, Expectorant, Sedative, Tonic.

PRECAUTIONS: A lingering aroma, often persists in clothes after they have been washed. Its aphrodisiac qualities are well known and should be used at your own peril! Perhaps best avoided in states of depression – it may lower mood even further.

MIND: A very relaxing oil, soothes nervous tension and anxiety – more sedative than uplifting. Reputedly helpful in dealing with obsessional attitudes and said to cut ties with the past. Could be used to comfort the dying since it helps to bring peace and acceptance.

BODY: Very useful to the genito-urinary system alleviating cystitis and should be massaged in the kidney region where it has a purifying and anti-inflammatory action.

Its aphrodisiac qualities can relieve sexual problems such as frigidity and impotence, perhaps dealing with the underlying anxiety. Its antispasmodic and tonic action on the body should encourage relaxation and a feeling of well being. Was once used to alleviate sex-transmitted diseases and may well have a cleansing action on the sexual organs. Could be useful in promoting vaginal secretions.

Also helpful with chest infections, sore throats and dry coughs which accompany bronchitis and lung infections. Very relaxing and aids sleep when catarrhal conditions present. Helps to stimulate the immune system and keep infection at bay.

May also treat heartburn (a burning sensation just below the ribcage) and could be helpful for diarrhoea due to its astringent properties.

EFFECT ON SKIN: Generally a balancing oil but particularly good for dry eczema as well as ageing and dehydrated skins. Gives a softening effect and makes a good neck cream mixed with cocoa butter. It relieves itching and inflammation and its antiseptic qualities may be helpful with acne, boils and infected wounds.

BLENDS: Basil, Benzoin, Black Pepper, Cypress, Frankincense, Geranium, Jasmine, Lavender, Lemon, Myrrh, Neroli, Palmarosa, Rose, Vetivert, Ylang Ylang.

SANTOLINA

Plant/Part	:	Shrub/Seeds
Latin Name	:	Santolina chamaecyparissias
Family	:	Compositae
Note	:	?
Planet	:	Mercury or Moon
Extraction	:	Distillation

AROMA: Almost like a spicy-apple.

FEATURES: Though also known as 'Lavender Cotton', it is not a Labiate, and is in fact, related to the daisy family. An evergreen, it grows to about two feet and has a white stem with cotton-like silver-grey hairy leaves and tiny yellow flowers. It is found in Italy, southern France and the Mediterranean countries though also cultivated in England. Survives intense heat and lack of water for long periods and the highest yield of oil is just before the flowering period.

HISTORY & MYTH: Credit goes to the Normans for introducing Santolina, amongst other things, into Britain. It was certainly a thriving plant in these isles by the 16th century and often grown as a hedging plant. The name Santolina stems from the Latin meaning 'saintly flax' which points to the high regard in which it was held.

It was used extensively in France as an insecticide where it is referred to as 'garde-robe' since it was placed in clothes cupboards and bed linen to keep the bugs away. A popular strewing herb and an ingredient of many European medicines mainly for its antispasmodic and vermifuge properties. Not produced as an oil on a large commercial scale.

CHEMICAL CONSTITUENTS: Borneol (Alcohol), Cineole (Ketone), Camphene, Cymene, Limonene, Myrcene, Phellandrene, Pinene, Sabinene, Terpinene, Terpinolene (Terpenes).

PROPERTIES: Antiphlogistic, Antispasmodic, Escharotic, Emmenagogue, Hepatic, Stimulant, Stomachic, Tonic, Vermifuge.

PRECAUTIONS: Might prove slightly toxic with prolonged use and could be a skin irritant. Best avoided in pregnancy.

MIND: Could have a simulating and refreshing effect on the mind.

BODY: Best effect appears to be as a vermifuge, expelling worms from the intestines. An excellent insect repellent and helpful for poisonous bites and stings.

Seems to clear obstructions from the liver, could be effective in cases of jaundice and cleanses the kidneys. Soothes gastric spasms and a general tonic to the digestive system.

May help with genital problems like leucorrhoea and said to regulate scanty periods.

Some benefit may be obtained for asthma and coughs.

EFFECT ON SKIN: Minimises itching especially where there is inflammation and helps to heal scabs. Said to have a clearing effect on ringworm, verrucae and warts.

BLENDS: Chamomile, Lavender, Mandarin, Orange.

SPEARMINT

Plant/Part	:	Herb/Flowering tops and leaves
Latin Name	:	Mentha spicata
Family	:	Labiatae
Note	:	Top
Planet	:	Venus
Extraction	:	Distillation

AROMA: Similar to Peppermint though slightly sweeter.

FEATURES: The wrinkled and spiked leaves give Spearmint its name. It reaches to about three feet and has purple flowers. There are of course, many varieties of mint and mostly all possess the same properties. Unlike Peppermint though, Spearmint does not contain Menthol. It originally grew in the Mediterranean region and North Africa but is now cultivated mainly in America, Asia and Britain.

HISTORY & MYTH: Spearmint was used as tonic and scent by the ancient Greeks who used it liberally in their bathwater. It had a reputation for curing sexually transmitted diseases like gonorrhoea which is just as well since it also found fame as an aphrodisiac. The Romans introduced Spearmint into Britain where it was mainly used to stop milk curdling. However, in medieval times it became a feature in oral hygiene and was used to heal sore gums and also for whitening the teeth.

CHEMICAL CONSTITUENTS: Carvone, Cineole (Ketones), Caryophyllene (Sesquiterpene), Limonene, Myrcene, Phellandrene (Terpenes).

PROPERTIES: Antipruritic, Antispasmodic, Carminative, Emmenagogue, Insecticide, Parturient, Restorative, Stimulant.

PRECAUTIONS: A sharp oil so total body massage may not be a good idea, unless a minute dosage is used. Massage in local areas may be preferable however. Possibility of irritating the eyes as well as sensitive skin. Best avoided in pregnancy. Could antidote homoeopathic remedies.

MIND: Stimulates a tired mind.

BODY: Helpful with digestive problems like vomiting, flatulence, constipation and diarrhoea. Seems to relax the stomach muscles, relieves hiccups and nausea. May help mitigate some of the effects of travel and sea sickness. Overall, a tonic to the digestive organs and stimulates the appetite.

Also said to release retention of urine and dissolves kidney stones apparently.

May have some effect on the reproductive system since it controls over abundance of breast milk as well as hardening of the breasts. In the same way, could well stem the flow of heavy periods and leucorrhoea. Said to promote easier labour during childbirth.

Also good for headaches, bad breath and sore gums.

EFFECT ON SKIN: The herb has been used for pruritus – a severe itching of the skin – and the oil may also provide relief. In a like manner may be helpful for sores and scabs.

BLENDS: Basil, Grapefruit, Linden Blossom, Rosemary.

TAGETES

Plant/Part	:	Shrub/Flowers and Leaves
Latin Name	:	Tagetes patula/glandulifera
Family	:	Compositae
Note	:	Top to Middle
Planet	:	Jupiter or Sun
Extraction	:	Distillation

AROMA: Sweet, fruity yet almost citrus-like.

FEATURES: The original Tagetes (T. erecta) was cultivated in North Africa though rumour has it that a Central American pedigree is more correct. However, it now mainly grown in France and referred to as 'French Marigold'. The deeply divided feathery leaves surround small carnation-like bright orange flowers. Its only after the full flowering stage that the oil is distilled.

HISTORY & MYTH: In Africa it was known as 'Khakibush' and was often seen hanging from native huts to deter the regular swarm of flies. It was also planted amongst tomatoes, potatoes and roses to dissuade eelworms from making a feast of the crops. All in all it seemed to be an effective larvicide and was also made into ointments to kill ravaging maggots in wounds. The roots and seeds have been found to be purgative, probably helping the rid the body of poisons.

Just after the Boer War, at the turn of the century, Australian troops brought the plant to their native land where the roots grew profusely. Used extensively in French perfumes.

CHEMICAL CONSTITUENTS: Tagetone (Ketone), Limonene, Ocimene (Terpenes).

PROPERTIES: Antimicrobe, Antiphlogistic, Antiseptic, Antispasmodic, Cytophylactic, Emollient, Fungicide, Insecticide, Hypotensive, Sedative.

PRECAUTIONS: A very powerful oil and should be used sparingly.

MIND: Said to clear thinking, relieve tension and promote a firmer hold on the emotions.

BODY: Its well known antimicrobe action is valuable for keeping disease carrying mosquitoes and flies at bay and possibly helping to keep a check on infected bites.

Said to be effective against ear infections, possibly improves the hearing and may sharpen the senses generally.

Seems to have an affinity with the respiratory system, dilates the bronchi facilitating flow of mucous and dislodges congestion. May also help relieve coughs.

Appears to have a reputation in easing aches and pains as well as sprains and strains.

Its sedative action could help to bring down high blood pressure.

EFFECT ON SKIN: A useful oil, it would seem, for dealing with skin infections particularly suppurations. Its healing effect on wounds and cuts is probably due to its ability to soothe inflammatory conditions. May also help to clear fungal infections.

BLENDS: Chamomile, Coriander, Frankincense, Geranium, Lavender, Lemon, Linden Blossom, Orange, Sandalwood, Tangerine, Ti-Tree, Ylang Ylang.

TANGERINE

Plant/Part	:	Fruit/Peel
Latin Name	:	Citrus reticulata
Family	:	Rutaceae
Note	:	Top to Middle
Planet	:	?
Extraction	:	Cold Expression

AROMA: Sweet, light and tangy.

FEATURES: Tangerine is from the same botanical source as Mandarin though represents a lower stage in the horticultural development of the fruit. Tends to be harvested earlier, around November rather than February and is a deeper orange, Mandarin being a little more yellow. The two fruits share a similar aroma though Tangerine is probably weaker, or more subtle. A native of China, the oil is largely produced in USA followed by Sicily. Incidentally, Tangerine does not have pips, Mandarin does.

HISTORY & MYTH: Tangerine was introduced into the USA from China via Europe. Sometimes known as 'Dancy Tangerine' after Colonel G L Dancy, who apparently first started growing the fruit from seedlings in the southern states of America, around 1871.

CHEMICAL CONSTITUENTS: Citronellol, Linalool (Alcohols), Citral (Aldehyde), Cadinene (Sesquiterpene), Limonene (Terpene).

PROPERTIES: Antiseptic, Antispasmodic, Cytophylactic, Sedative, Stomachic, Tonic.

PRECAUTIONS: Could be phototoxic and care should be taken not to expose the skin to strong sunlight after treatment.

MIND: Said to have an almost hypnotic effect. In any event may well be helpful with stress and tension due to its soothing action on the nervous system.

BODY: Its medicinal properties are apparently close to Orange, which may go for Mandarin as well. Certainly all three seem to have an effect on the digestive system, dealing with all manner of gastric complaints like flatulence, diarrhoea, constipation as well as stimulating flow of bile, thus helping to digest fats.

A tonic to the vascular system particularly the peripheral circulation which nourishes the veins and arteries in the extremities, therefore activating tired and aching limbs.

A popular massage choice in pregnancy since it is useful for the vitamin C content.

EFFECT ON SKIN: Brings back colour to pale skins due to its re-energising action on the blood. A useful skin tonic and could help smooth out stretch marks particularly when blended with Lavender and Neroli.

BLENDS: Basil, Bergamot, Chamomile, Clary Sage, Frankincense, Geranium, Grapefruit, Lavender, Lemon, Lime, Neroli, Orange, Rose.

TARRAGON

Plant/Part	:	Herb/Flowering plant
Latin Name	:	Artemisia dracunculus
Family	:	Compositae
Note	:	Top
Planet	:	Mars
Extraction	:	Distillation

AROMA: Herby, anisic and spicy.

FEATURES: Tarragon thrives best near rivers and streams. Its woody stem reaches to about three feet and has widely spaced, narrow olive green leaves with tiny white/grey flowers. Though originally from the Middle East, the oil was for some time obtained from Russia though latterly superseded by the French variety which is of better quality reputedly.

HISTORY & MYTH: 'Estragon', as it is sometimes called, was introduced into Spain by the conquering Moors and was well known in Britain by the 16th century. The name is derived from the Arabic 'Tharkhoum' and the Latin 'Dracunculus' meaning little dragon probably because its root seems to coil up like a dragon. In any event, it was useful for treating snake bites and those of mad dogs.

A myth goes that the herb was also named after Artemesia, Greek goddess of the Hunt and Childbirth. It is a very popular culinary herb, being an ingredient of tarragon vinegar, tartare sauce and salt-free diets. It is rich in vitamins A and C and in the past has been used to treat scurvy whereas the root was found to be useful in toothache. There is also a past connection in clearing cancers. Another ingredient of French perfumes.

CHEMICAL CONSTITUENTS: Methylchavicol (Phenol), Ocimene, Phellandrene (Terpenes).

PROPERTIES: Antirheumatic, Antiseptic, Antispasmodic, Aperitif, Carminative, Digestive, Diuretic, Emmenagogue, Laxative, Stimulant, Stomachic, Vermifuge.

PRECAUTIONS: Some risk of toxicity with prolonged use and should be avoided in pregnancy.

MIND: May get things moving again, banishing apathy and boredom – instilling incentive.

BODY: Could be helpful with conditions of a chronic nature and generally seems to have a cleansing effect. This may be partly due to its diuretic properties, thereby clearing the kidneys and helpful where there is difficulty in urinating. At the same time loosening build-up of uric acid, a contributory cause of arthritis.

May also have a soothing and pain relieving action on rheumatism and neuralgia.

A pronounced effect on the digestive system when it feels fragile, weak and seething! It stimulates appetite and to some extent controls nausea, belching and hiccups. Acts as a laxative and aids secretion of bile, promoting digestion of fats.

Quite effective on the reproductive system by regulating erratic periods and calming menstrual pain. Could have some influence or infertility.

EFFECT ON SKIN: Useful in treating weeping wounds.

BLENDS: Angelica, Carrot Seed, Chamomile, Clary Sage, Fir, Juniper, Lavender, Lime, Pine, Mandarin, Rosewood, Verbena.

TEREBINTH

Plant/Part	:	Tree
Latin Name	:	Pinus sylvestris Pinus palustris Pinus martima etc
Family	:	Pinaceae
Note	:	Middle
Planet	:	Mars
Extraction	:	Distillation and Solvent Extraction

AROMA: Fresh, similar to Pine, but more resinous.

FEATURES: Turpentine, a resin obtained from the many species of conifer tree, furnishes the essential oil upon distillation. Owing to demand, large amounts are produced, the chief sources being France and the USA.

HISTORY & MYTH: The Greek medics Hippocrates and Galen used Terebinth in liniments probably for infected wounds. More recently, in the last century, large scale production began in the USA since the southern states had enormous forests of conifers. The oil has been used as a solvent – thinning paints and varnishes – as well as an illuminant and in the production of lamp black. The resin was also employed in the American naval industry to repair wooden ships and rigging.

 During the American Civil War supplies were cut off from the southern states and other sources from the pines of Sierra Nevada in California provided the North. This industry thrived for a while but declined after the southern routes opened again. These days Terebinth is often used in pharmaceuticals.

CHEMICAL CONSTITUENTS: Camphene, Carene, Dipentene, Myrcene, Phellandrene, Terpinolene, Pinene (Terpenes).

PROPERTIES: Analgesic, Antipruritic, Antirheumatic, Antiseptic, Antispasmodic, Balsamic, Cicatrisant, Diuretic, Haemostatic, Insecticide, Parasiticide, Rubefacient, Vermifuge.

PRECAUTIONS: Some experts say that this oil should not be used in massage as skin sensitisation is a probability. It should in any event, be avoided by people suffering from epilepsy.

MIND: ?

BODY: Probably most beneficial to the muscular and skeletal system due to its rubefacient and analgesic action. Could be helpful with rheumatic pain, gout, neuralgia, sciatica and muscular aches generally.

Releases phlegm particularly in cases of bronchitis and helpful with pulmonary haemorrhages as well as general problems of the respiratory tract. May treat whooping cough and sore throats.

Valuable antiseptic of the urinary tract, easing cystitis, oligaria (insufficient urine) and urethritis (inflammation of the urethra). Also said to dissolve gall stones. Helpful with leucorrhoea and infections of the genital tract following childbirth.

Beneficial to the digestion, being effective with chronic constipation, flatulence and colitis. Also said to clear the intestines of parasites.

May also stem flow of blood as in nosebleeding and Valnet says haemophilia.

EFFECT ON SKIN: Could well be beneficial to infected wounds.

BLENDS: Benzoin, Camphor, Cypress, Eucalyptus, Ginger, Lavender, Origanum, Rosemary, Thyme.

THYME

Plant/Part	:	Herb/Flowers and leaves
Latin Name	:	Thymus vulgaris
Family	:	Labiatae
Note	:	Top to Middle
Planet	:	Venus
Extraction	:	Distillation

AROMA: A rather sweet and strongly herbal fragrance.

FEATURES: The many species of Thyme are derived from the original Wild Thyme (Thymus serphyllum), native to southern Europe. These days Thyme is cultivated in Gt. Britain, America and France. The stems reach to about eight inches bearing small elliptical greenish grey leaves and white or purple/pink flowers. White Thyme Oil is a purified version of Red Thyme Oil.

HISTORY & MYTH: Thyme has a long history in the ancient pharmacopoeia. An ingredient of perfume too since the name is derived from the Greek 'thymos' meaning 'to perfume'. It was also used as incense, burnt at the altars of Greek deities and a myth goes that it was born from the copious tears of Helen of Troy. The Egyptians thought it effective in embalming probably due to its strong preservative properties.

Credit goes to the Romans for introducing the herb to the rest of Europe. During the Age of Chivalry, it was given to jousting Knights for courage and in the later Middle Ages its strong antiseptic quality played an important part in the judicial system. Sprigs of Thyme were carried by judges into their courtrooms to ward off infection. It was also used for such serious diseases as paralysis, multiple sclerosis, leprosy and muscular atrophy.

CHEMICAL CONSTITUENTS: Borneol, Linalool (Alcohols), Carvacrol, Thymol (Phenols), Caryophyllene (Sesquiterpene), Cymene, Terpinene (Terpenes).

PROPERTIES: Antimicrobe, Antirheumatic, Antiseptic, Antispasmodic, Antiputrefactive, Antivenomous, Aperitif, Aphrodisiac, Bactericide, Bechic, Cardiac, Carminative, Cicatrisant, Diuretic, Emmenagogue, Expectorant, Hypertensive, Insecticide, Stimulant, Tonic, Vermifuge.

PRECAUTIONS: A very potent oil, one of the strongest antiseptics and toxicity is possible with prolonged use. Inhalations may be preferable to massage or baths since could irritate the skin though the mucous membranes may be susceptible too. Not to be used in cases of high blood pressure, nor in pregnancy.

MIND: Strengthens the nerves and activates the brain cells thereby aiding memory and concentration. Revives low spirits, feelings of exhaustion and combats depression. Said also to release mental blockages and trauma.

BODY: Fortifies the lungs when treating colds, coughs and sore throats particularly tonsillitis, laryngitis, pharyngitis, bronchitis, whooping cough and asthma. Rather warming and helps to eliminate phlegm.

Basically stimulates action of white corpuscles and helps the body fight disease and deters the spread of germs. Beneficial to the immune system.

Good for the circulation and raises low blood pressure. May be used for rheumatism, gout, arthritis and sciatica since its stimulating effect and diuretic action facilitates the removal of uric acid. When used in a compress can reduce painful arthritic swelling. May stop nosebleeding.

A digestive stimulant, intestinal antiseptic and particularly good in gastric infections, expels worms and eases dyspepsia. Helpful with sluggish digestion and wind as well as headaches resulting from gastric complaints. As a urinary antiseptic, may be helpful with cystitis.

Seems to allay menstrual difficulties such as scanty periods and leucorrhoea. Said to be helpful in childbirth – speeding delivery and expelling afterbirth – a cleansing action which could help in cases of miscarriage as well.

EFFECT ON SKIN: A tonic for the scalp and may be effective with dandruff and hair loss. Often helpful with wounds and sores as well as dermatitis, boils and carbuncles.

BLENDS: Bergamot, Cedarwood, Chamomile, Juniper, Lemon, Niaouli, Mandarin, Melissa, Rosemary, Ti-Tree.

TI-TREE

Plant/Part	:	Tree/Leaf
Latin Name	:	Melaleuca alternifolia
Family	:	Myrtaceae
Note	:	Top
Planet	:	?
Extraction	:	Distillation

AROMA: Fresh and sanitary, rather pungent.

FEATURES: A very useful essential oil, sometimes spelt 'Tea-Tree' but is not connected to the cup that cheers – that is 'Camellia Thea'. M. Alternifolia is a small tree from New South Wales similar to Cypress. It grows to about twenty feet and thrives in marshy areas though now cultivated in plantations. Has great vitality, continuing to flourish even when chopped down and is ready for cutting again after two years. The oil is only produced in Australia.

HISTORY & MYTH: The Australian Aborigines have long recognised the virtues of Ti-Tree. When the rest of the world thought it was just a weed, they used the leaves to cure infected wounds. It was introduced into Europe around 1927 and its excellent antiseptic quality was quickly noted. Indeed, the English settlers followed the example set by the Aborigines and found the leaves useful when medical supplies were unobtainable.

Ti-Tree is a new addition to Aromatherapy though its popularity has risen quickly due to its immuno-stimulant effect. Active research has been carried out in Australia, America and France on its anti-infectious and anti-fungal power especially in treating a variety of skin conditions.

During World War Two, it was included in military aid kits in tropical areas as well as in munition factories for skin injuries. Used frequently in surgical and dental practise as well as in soaps, deodorants, disinfectants and air fresheners.

CHEMICAL CONSTITUENTS: Terpinenol (Alcohol), Cineole (Ketone), Cymene, Pinene, Terpinene (Terpenes).

PROPERTIES: Antibiotic, Antipruritic, Antiseptic, Antiviral, Bactericide, Balsamic, Cicatrisant, Cordial, Expectorant, Fungicide, Insecticide, Stimulant, Sudorific.

PRECAUTIONS: May cause irritation on sensitive areas of skin.

MIND: Refreshing and revitalising especially after shock.

BODY: Its most important usage is to help the immune system fight off infectious diseases. Activates the white corpuscles to form a defence against invading organisms and helps to shorten the duration of illness. A strongly antiseptic oil and sweats toxins out of the body. Indicated for influenza, cold sores, catarrh and could treat glandular fever as well as gingivitis. Though not offering a cure, could be of service in helping to strengthen the immune system with A.I.D.'s patients. Naturally this is best done in co-operation with qualified medical personnel.

A course of massage with Ti-Tree before an operation will help to fortify the body. Also effective in reducing post operative shock. Its strong antiviral and germicidal properties are useful in repeated infections, post viral debility and bestows vigour in convalescence.

Its fungicidal properties help clear vaginal thrush and is of value with genital infections generally. Also a urinary tract antiseptic, alleviating problems such as cystitis. Gives relief to genital and anal pruritus as well as general itching from chicken pox to rashes caused by insect bites.

Said to give some protection against X-ray therapy in breast cancer. It will apparently reduce scarring when applied before treatment as the protective film will guard against very deep penetration of the X rays.

Helps to ease otitis, a middle ear infection which is often linked to ailing tonsils. May also ease inflammation of the intestines such as enteritis and casts out intestinal parasites.

EFFECT ON SKIN: Very cleansing – reducing pus in infected wounds as well as boils and carbuncles. Seems to clear spots and blemishes caused by chicken pox and shingles. Useful with burns, sores, sunburn, ringworm, warts, tinea, herpes and athletes foot. Helpful with dry conditions of the scalp as well as dandruff.

BLENDS: Cinnamon, Clove, Cypress, Eucalyptus, Ginger, Lavender, Lemon, Mandarin, Orange, Rosemary, Thyme.

VERBENA

Plant/Part	:	Shrub/Stalks and leaves
Latin Name	:	Lippia citriodora
Family	:	Verbenaceae
Note	:	Top
Planet	:	Venus
Extraction	:	Distillation

AROMA: Like a sweet lemon.

FEATURES: A small bush with abundant leaves, rather delicate and sensitive to frosts. It has light green, slightly crinkled leaves with pale pink flowers. Brought to Europe in the 18th century from South America and much of the essential oil is obtained from Algeria and Spain. Sometimes confused with Vervain (Verbena Officinalis) or the exotic Verbena, Litsea Cubeba.

HISTORY & MYTH: 'Lippia' was named after a European doctor and botanist born in 1678 and 'Citriodora' stems from the citrus aroma. Also referred to as Lemon Verbena and began to grace English gardens in the 18th century. A popular beverage drink on the Continent, flavouring liqueurs as well.

Witches cashed in on its reputation as an aphrodisiac and used it in their love potions. Often included in pot-pourri to guard against germs, along with Cinnamon, Clove, Juniper, Lemon, Lavender, Thyme and Sandalwood. The herb was once applied to inflamed eyes and mouth sores. These days the oil is used in soaps and perfumes though the low yield of essential oil makes for a high price.

CHEMICAL CONSTITUENTS: Borneol, Geraniol, Linalool, Nerol (Alcohols), Citral (Aldehyde, Ketone), Dipentene, Limonene, Myrcene (Terpenes).

PROPERTIES: Antiseptic, Antispasmodic, Aphrodisiac, Digestive, Emollient, Febrifuge, Hepatic, Insecticide, Sedative, Stomachic, Tonic.

PRECAUTIONS: It seems that recent pharmacological tests have proven this oil to be phototoxic and a strong skin sensitiser. It may well be a good idea not to include Verbena in massage.

MIND: Famed for banishing depression due to its tonic and soothing effect on the parasympathetic nervous system. It has a relaxing, refreshing and yet uplifting action on the emotions and helps deal with stress.

BODY: Works on the digestive system especially controlling stomach spasm and cramp, nausea, indigestion and flatulence. Stimulates the appetite and has an action on bile aiding digestion of fats. A cooling action on the liver mitigates inflammation and infection, as in cirrhosis, and could be beneficial in cases of alcoholism.

Seems to be of some help to the respiratory system possibly for bronchitis as well as nasal and sinus congestion. Said to avert convulsions and soothes asthmatic coughs.

Calms heart palpitations (tachycardia) and may deal with nervous insomnia.

Its reputation as an aphrodisiac probably stems from its ability to calm underlying tension.

EFFECT ON SKIN: Appears to soften the skin and keep down puffiness. Could also be a useful hair tonic.

BLENDS: Basil, Bergamot, Chamomile, Geranium, Grapefruit, Lavender, Lime, Neroli, Palmarosa, Rose, Rosemary, Ylang Ylang.

VETIVERT

Plant/Part	:	Grass/Root
Latin Name	:	Andropogon muricatus
Family	:	Gramineae
Note	:	Base
Planet	:	?
Extraction	:	Distillation

AROMA: Deep, smoky and earthy fragrance.

FEATURES: A wild grass mainly found in tropical areas such as India, Tahiti, Java and Haiti. The little that has been cultivated in the Americas was sold principally as scent sachets. Since the oil is difficult to separate from water, the yield of oil is generally low. The older the root, the better the oil which also improves with age.

HISTORY & MYTH: Known as 'the oil of tranquillity' due to its calming action. In Calcutta, awnings, blinds and sunshades were made out of Vetivert grass otherwise known as 'Kus-Kus'. Sprinkled with water in the hot weather they gave out an exquisite scent. The powdered root, used in sachets, protected Indian muslin from moths and insects. In Java, the root has been used for centuries in weaving mats and thatching huts whereas the natives in Haiti thought the grassy parts better for their thatched roofs.

A famous European perfume called 'Mousseline des Indes' contained Vetivert, along with Sandalwood, Benzoin, Thyme and Rose. Indeed, it is often used as a fixative in perfumes. Before the First World War Java exported large quantities of dried Vetivert root to Europe for distillation, but due to crowded shipping lanes, Java begun to distil plant material locally where it was referred to as 'Akar wangi'.

CHEMICAL CONSTITUENTS: Benzoic (Acid), Vetiverol (Alcohol), Furfurol (Aldehyde), Vetivone (Ketone), Vetivene (Sesquiterpene).

PROPERTIES: Antiseptic, Aphrodisiac, Nervine, Sedative, Tonic.

PRECAUTIONS: ?

MIND: A calming oil and a reputed panacea for stress and tension. Useful just before a lecture or a visit to the dentist – seems to settle the nerves. Also could help people who feel out of balance and need grounding. Deeper psychological problems may also respond especially where there is too much sensitivity and openness.

BODY: Its balancing effect on the central nervous system instills a more centred feeling and may be useful in helping people ease off tranquillisers. Said to cleanse the aura – the energy field around the body – and to strengthen the auric shield which can be instrumental in keeping out disease.

Despite its sedative action, very helpful in cases of mental and physical exhaustion. It revitalises the body by fortifying the red blood corpuscles crucial in transporting oxygen to all parts of the system.

Increased blood flow could alleviate muscular aches and pains and said to be useful in cases of rheumatism and arthritis.

Reputedly a tonic to the reproductive system and its relaxing quality seems to have some effect on tension underlying sexual problems.

Generally helps to restore the body back to health, not least through its ability to promote sleep, helpful in cases of insomnia.

EFFECT ON SKIN: May have a healing effect on acne.

BLENDS: Benzoin, Frankincense, Galbanum, Geranium, Grapefruit, Jasmine, lavender, Patchouli, Rose, Rosewood, Sandalwood, Violet, Ylang Ylang.

VIOLET

Plant/Part	:	Flower/leaves
Latin Name	:	Viola odorata
Family	:	Violaceae
Note	:	Middle to Base
Planet	:	Venus
Extraction	:	Enfleurage

AROMA: Dry, sweet and somewhat hay-like.

FEATURES: There are numerous species of Violet which grow all over the world though a great deal of the essential oil comes from France and Egypt. The plant favours damp woodlands and shady places. It has long stalks and heart shaped dark green leaves with delicate, blue/violet flowers.

HISTORY & MYTH: The Violet was a symbol of fertility in Ancient Greece and the adopted emblem of Athens. Revered highly by the Romans who planted it amongst their garlic and onions! It was used as a cosmetic among the Celts who infused the flowers in goat's milk as a complexion aid. The Anglo Saxons however, thought it a good remedy against evil spirits.

Though a favourite perfume of Marie Antoinette it did not deter Napoleon from adopting it as his party's insignia! Later in the 19th century, hot compresses of violet leaves were applied to malignant tumours in an effort to relieve pain. More recently candied sweets – 'Violet Plantes' – were used for chest problems. Two types were used in the perfume industry – Parma and Victoriana. Parma was preferred for its scent but Victoriana, a hardier species, became popular at the turn of the century.

CHEMICAL CONSTITUENTS: Salicylic (Acid), Benzyl (Alcohol), . Parmone (Ketone), Eugenol (Phenol).

PROPERTIES: Antiseptic, Aphrodisiac, Bechic, Diuretic, Emetic, Expectorant, Laxative, Pectoral, Sedative.

PRECAUTIONS: ?

MIND: Its sedative properties overcome insomnia and banish feelings of anger and anxiety. Reputedly restores the bonds of friendship.

BODY: Violet has an affinity with the kidneys and tends to exert a purging effect on urine, therefore helpful with cystitis particularly where there is sharp pain in the lower back. May also help to disperse general congestion in the body and has mild laxative properties. Will also induce vomiting. Often acts as a liver decongestant too and could be helpful with jaundice, as well as clearing hangovers!

Has a beneficial effect on the respiratory tract and could be helpful with irritating coughs, whooping cough and particularly where there are breathing problems, i.e. shortness of breath.

Soothes inflammation of the throat, hoarseness and pleurisy. Dissolves mucous and expels catarrh.

Seems to alleviate congestion of the head, dealing with headaches, giddiness and fits apparently and may be of service in cases of epilepsy.

Supposedly a strong aphrodisiac, beneficial to sexual problems, reputedly restoring libido. Possibly of assistance with menopausal symptoms such as irritability and hot flushes.

Also said to have some pain killing properties and may ease rheumatism, fibrositis and gout.

EFFECT ON SKIN: A strong antiseptic and useful in treating wounds, bruises, congested skin, swellings and inflammation. Said to heal cracked nipples.

BLENDS: Benzoin, Citronella, Frankincense, Grapefruit, Jasmine, Lavender, Lemon, Orange, Sandalwood, Verbena, Rose.

YARROW

Plant/Part	:	Bush/Flowering heads
Latin Name	:	Achillea millefolium
Family	:	Compositae
Note	:	Top
Planet	:	Venus
Extraction	:	Distillation

AROMA: Slightly sweet and spicy.

FEATURES: A familiar hedgerow bush found along country lanes principally in Europe, Western Asia and North America. It grows to about three feet and has fern-like, feathery leaves with pink and white flowers which are bonded in clusters on tough angular stems. Also known as Milfoil, referring to its feathery appearance.

HISTORY & MYTH: A plant of divination and used as a charm in Scotland. Credited with powers to ward off evil spirits and secreted in churches to this effect. Young maidens were also hopeful about its magical effects and placed it under their pillows to dream of true love. A myth goes that Achilles during the wars with Troy tended his soldiers' wounds with Yarrow. Similarly the Anglo-Saxons healed wounds inflicted with iron. Interestingly, Yarrow is also known as the Military herb.

Its reputation grew as having an all-healing action and was used for a variety of ailments throughout the ages from lung cancer and diabetes to severe colds and as snuff to cause nosebleeds – a blood letting technique no doubt. The Swedes add it to their beer for a more rousing effect.

CHEMICAL CONSTITUENTS: Borneol (Alcohol), Cineole (Ketone), Azuline (Sesquiterpene), Limonene, Pinene (Terpenes).

PROPERTIES: Antiphlogistic, Antiseptic, Antispasmodic, Astringent, Cholagogue, Diuretic, Expectorant, Febrifuge, Stimulant, Tonic.

PRECAUTIONS: Prolonged use may cause headaches and irritate sensitive skins. Might be too potent to use in pregnancy.

MIND: Possibly helpful when spirits are low.

BODY: A general fortifier since Yarrow acts directly on the bone marrow and stimulates blood renewal. It is a tonic to the vascular system improving circulatory disorders such as varicose veins and haemorrhoids.

An excellent oil for the female reproductive system since it seems to have an hormonal action. Deals with irregular menstruation, especially heavy periods, menopausal problems, inflammation of the ovaries, prolapse of the uterus and fibroids.

Stimulates secretion of gastric and intestinal glands and improves sluggish digestion. Balances the nervous component of digestion, improving absorption and digestive secretions, helpful for colic and flatulence. Stimulates bile aiding digestion of fats and encourages appetite. Its astringent properties also help to stem diarrhoea.

Helpful for feverish colds, congestion in the head and promotes perspiration by opening the sweat glands encouraging a cleansing and cooling action.

Said to have a balancing force on the flow of urine, useful with stangury (retention of urine) as well as involuntary discharge of urine, i.e. bed-wetting.

Its pain relieving properties may be helpful with back ache, rheumatic pain and headaches.

Mosquitos, it is said, find it less than pleasing.

EFFECT ON SKIN: Healing is said to be slow but sure where inflamed wounds, cuts, chapped hands and ulcers are concerned. Its astringent properties seem to balance oily complexions and it is also known as a tonic and conditioner for the scalp. A stimulating action on hair growth may deal with falling hair and even baldness.

BLENDS: Angelica, Clary Sage, Juniper, Lemon, Melissa, Rosemary, Tarragon, Verbena.

YLANG-YLANG

Plant/Part	:	Tree/Flowers
Latin Name	:	Cananga odorata
Family	:	Anonaceae
Note	:	Middle to Base
Planet	:	Venus?
Extraction	:	Distillation

AROMA: Sweet, floral, exotic and heavy.

FEATURES: Varieties of pink, mauve and yellow flowers grow on this small tropical tree though the finer oil is distilled from the yellow blooms. The first oil drawn from the flowers is the best quality though subsequent yields have similar therapeutic features, only the perfume is less refined. It is then known as Cananga. A semi-wild tree with brittle wood and is found in the south sea islands notably the Seychelles, Mauritius, Tahiti as well as the Philippines – where the best oil comes from apparently.

HISTORY & MYTH: This 'flower of flowers' derives from the Malay 'Alang-ilang' indicating the way the flowers hang. The tree is apparently 'a crown in the East' and is also known as 'the perfume tree'. In the South Seas, women dress their hair with essential oil of Ylang Ylang in a mixture of coconut oil. Indeed, it was once used as an ingredient of hair preparations in Europe, known as Macasser oil, hence the anti-macassers on the backs of armchairs to stop greasy stains.

A lovely custom in Indonesia sees beds spread with these petals on wedding nights. No doubt honouring the aphrodisiac qualities for which the perfume is famed. Up until 1900, the Philippines had world trade monopoly on what was sometimes called 'the poor man's Jasmine'. It is however used extensively in classy perfumes.

CHEMICAL CONSTITUENTS: Benzoic (Acid), Farnesol, Geranoil, Linalool (Alcohols), Benzyl acetate (Ester), Eugenol, Safrole (Phenols), Cadinene (Sesquiterpene), Pinene (Terpene).

PROPERTIES: Antidepressant, Antiseptic, Aphrodisiac, Hypotensive, Sedative.

PRECAUTIONS: Excessive use may lead to headaches and nausea. Could possibly irritate sensitive skins and indicated against use on inflammatory skin conditions and dermatitis.

MIND: Excellent for excitable conditions regulating adrenaline flow and relaxing the nervous system, resulting in a feeling of joy. Could well ease feelings of anger, anxiety, shock, panic and fear.

BODY: Its reputed ability to balance the hormones makes it valuable for problems associated with the reproductive system. Principally, a tonic to the womb and could well be helpful after a caesarian birth instilling a feeling of warmth and togetherness. Also said to keep the breasts firm.

Its antidepressant and aphrodisiac qualities are well known in helping with sexual problems such as impotence and frigidity.

Particularly useful with rapid breathing (hyperpnoea) and rapid heartbeat (tachycardia) and its sedative properties could help bring down high blood pressure. Altogether has a relaxing effect on the nervous system though prolonged use may create an opposite effect.

Its antiseptic nature seems to have a beneficial action on intestinal infections.

EFFECT ON SKIN: A versatile oil, having a balancing action on sebum so making it effective on both oily and dry skins. Also has a tonic and stimulating effect on the scalp promoting a more luxurious hair growth.

BLENDS: Bergamot, Citronella, Grapefruit, Jasmine, lavender, Lemon, Melissa, Neroli, Orange, Patchouli, Rose, Rosewood, Sandalwood, Verbena.

Glossary

Anaesthetic: Loss of sensation – pain relieving.
Cinnamon, Clove, Peppermint,

Analgesic: Pain relieving.
Basil, Bay, Bergamot, Birch, Black Pepper, Cajuput, Camphor, Chamomile, Clove, Coriander, Eucalyptus, Galbanum, Geranium, Ginger, Lavandin, Lavender, Marjoram, Niaouli, Nutmeg, Origanum, Peppermint, Pimento, Rosemary, Terebinth.

Anaphrodisiac: Diminishing sexual desire.
Marjoram.

Antiacid: Combating acid in the body.
Lemon.

Antiallergenic: Reduces symptoms of allergy.
Chamomile, Melissa.

Antibiotic: Combats infection in the body.
Garlic, Ti-Tree.

Anticoagulant: Prevents blood from clotting.
Geranium.

Anticonvulsive: Controlling convulsions.
Chamomile, Clary Sage, Lavender.

Antidepressant: Uplifting, counteracting melancholy.
Basil, Bergamot, Citronella, Clary Sage, Geranium, Grapefruit, Jasmine, Lavender, Lemongrass, Litsea Cubeba, Melissa, Neroli, Orange, Patchouli, Petitgrain, Pimento, Rose, Rosemary, Rosewood, Ylang Ylang.

Antidontalgic: Relieving toothache.
Cajuput, Cinnamon, Clove, Nutmeg, Peppermint, Pimento.

Antiemetic: Reduces vomiting.
Aniseed, Anise-Star, Black Pepper, Chamomile, Cinnamon, Clove, Fennel, Ginger, Nutmeg.

Antigalactagogue: Impedes flow of milk.
Peppermint, Sage.

Antimicrobe: Reducing microbes.
Myrrh, Tagetes, Thyme.

Antineuralgic: Reducing nerve pain.
Bay, Cajuput, Clove, Lemon.

Antiphlogistic: Reducing inflammation.
Celery, Chamomile, Clary Sage, Eucalyptus, Fennel, Guaiacwood, Immortelle, Lavender, Myrrh, Patchouli, Peppermint, Pine, Rose, Sandalwood, Santolina, Tagetes, Yarrow.

Antiputrefactive: Delays decomposition of animal/vegetable matter.
Cinnamon, Thyme.

Antipruritic: Prevents itching.
Chamomile, Lemon, Spearmint, Terebinth, Ti-Tree

Antirheumatic: Helps to relieve rheumatism.
Cajuput, Celery, Chamomile, Cypress, Eucalyptus, Garlic, Guaiacwood, Hyssop, Juniper, Lemon, Lavender, Niaouli, Origanum, Pine, Rosemary, Sage, Tarragon, Terebinth, Thyme.

Antislcerotic: Prevents hardening of tissue due to chronic inflammation.
Garlic, Lemon.

Antiscorbutic: Helps with prevention of scurvy.
Fir, Ginger, Lemon, Lime.

Antiseptic: Helps to prevent tissue degeneration and controls infection.
Basil, Bergamot, Birch, Black Pepper, Cajuput, Camphor, Cedarwood, Chamomile, Cinnamon, Clary Sage, Clove, Cypress, Eucalyptus, Fennel, Fir, Frankincense, Garlic, Geranium, Ginger, Hyssop, Jasmine, Juniper, Lavender, Lemon, Lemongrass, Lime, Marjoram, Myrrh, Myrtle, Neroli, Niaouli, Nutmeg, Origanum, Palmarosa, Parsley, Peppermint, Pine, Rose, Rosemary, Rosewood, Sage, Sandalwood, Tagetes, Terebinth, Ti-Tree, Thyme, Verbena, Vetivert, Yarrow.

Antispasmodic: Relieves cramp.
Angelica, Aniseed, Basil, Bay, Bergamot, Black Pepper, Cajuput, Camphor, Caraway, Cardamum, Chamomile, Clary Sage, Clove, Coriander, Dill, Eucalyptus, Fennel, Ginger, Jasmine, Juniper, Hyssop, Lavender, Linden Blossom, Mandarin, Marjoram, Neroli, Nutmeg, Orange, Origanum, Parsley, Peppermint, Petitgrain, Rose, Rosemary, Sage,

Sandalwood, Spearmint, Tagetes, Tangerine, Terebinth, Thyme, Verbena, Yarrow.

Antisudorific: Reduces sweating.
Clary Sage, Cypress, Sage.

Antivenomous: Neutralises poison.
Basil, Thyme.

Antiviral: Controlling virus organisms.
Elemi, Eucalyptus, Garlic, Immortelle, Lavender, Lavender Spike, Lime, Palmarosa, Ti-Tree.

Aperitif: Encouraging appetite.
Bay, Caraway, Cardamom, Clove, Fennel, Ginger, Nutmeg, Origanum, Sage, Thyme, Tarragon.

Aphrodisiac: Exciting sexual desire.
Angelica, Aniseed, Basil, Black Pepper, Cardamum, Celery, Cinnamon, Clary Sage, Clove, Cumin, Ginger, Guaiacwood, Jasmine, Juniper, Nutmeg, Neroli, Parsley, Patchouli, Pimento, Rose, Rosewood, Sandalwood, Thyme, Verbena, Vetivert, Violet, Ylang Ylang.

Astringent: Contracts, tightens and binds tissues.
Bay, Benzoin, Birch, Caraway, Cedarwood, Cypress, Frankincense, Geranium, Guaiacwood, Hyssop, Immortelle, Juniper, Lemon, Lime, Myrrh, Myrtle, Patchouli, Peppermint, Rose, Rosemary, Sage, Sandalwood, Yarrow.

Bacteriacide: Combating bacteria.
Basil, Cumin, Elemi, Garlic, Eucalyptus, Immortelle, Lavender, Lemon, Lemongrass, Lime, Myrrh, Myrtle, Neroli, Niaouli, Palmarosa, Rose, Rosewood, Ti-Tree.

Balsamic: Healing, soothing and softening phlegm.
Cajuput, Clary Sage, Elemi, Eucalyptus, Guaiacwood, Myrrh, Niaouli, Pine, Terebinth, Ti-Tree.

Bechic: Eases coughs.
Ginger, Hyssop, Linden Blossom, Origanum, Sandalwood, Thyme.

Cardiac: Stimulating effect upon the heart.
Aniseed, Black Pepper, Caraway, Camphor, Cinnamon, Hyssop, Nutmeg, Thyme.

Carminative: Expulsion of gas from intestines.
Angelica, Aniseed, Anise-Star, Basil, Bergamot, Black Pepper, Caraway,

Cardamum, Carrot Seed, Celery, Chamomile, Cinnamon, Clove, Coriander, Cumin, Dill, Fennel, Galbanum, Ginger, Hyssop, Juniper, Lemon, Lemongrass, Marjoram, Melissa, Myrtle, Nutmeg, Orange, Origanum, Parsley, Peppermint, Pimento, Rosemary, Spearmint, Tarragon, Thyme.

Caustic: Burning.
Clove.

Cephalic: Stimulating and clearing the mind.
Basil, Cardamum, Hyssop, Marjoram, Peppermint, Rosemary, Rosewood.

Cholagogue: Increases bile production.
Bay, Chamomile, Garlic, Immortelle, Lavender, Peppermint, Rose, Rosemary, Yarrow.

Cicatrisant: Helping formation of scar tissue.
Bergamot, Cajuput, Chamomile, Clove, Cypress, Eucalyptus, Frankincense, Garlic, Geranium, Hyssop, Juniper, Lavender, Lavandin, Lemon, Niaouli, Patchouli, Rosemary, Sage, Terebinth, Ti-Tree.

Cordial: A tonic to the heart.
Benzoin, Bergamot, Lavender, Marjoram, Melissa, Neroli, Peppermint, Rosemary, Ti-Tree.

Cytophylactic: Encouraging growth of skin cells.
Carrot Seed, Frankincense, Geranium, Immortelle, Lavender, Mandarin, Palmarosa, Neroli, Rose, Tagetes, Tangerine.

Decongestant: Releasing nasal mucous.
Cajuput, Eucalyptus, Garlic, Lavender, Lavender Spike, Linden Blossom, Niaouli, Peppermint, Pine.

Deodorant: Destroying odour.
Benzoin, Bergamot, Citronella, Clary Sage, Coriander, Cypress, Eucalyptus, Geranium, Lavender, Lemongrass, Myrrh, Neroli, Patchouli, Pine, Rosewood, Petitgrain.

Depurative: Purifying the blood.
Birch, Caraway, Carrot Seed, Coriander, Cumin, Eucalyptus, Juniper, Lemon, Parsley, Rose, Sage.

Detoxicant: Neutralising toxic substances.
Black Pepper, Fennel, Frankincense, Juniper, Lavender.

Digestive: Aiding digestion.
Aniseed, Basil, Bergamot, Black Pepper, Caraway, Cardamum, Chamo-

mile, Clary Sage, Cumin, Dill, Lemongrass, Mandarin, Marjoram, Melissa, Neroli, Orange, Parsley, Rosemary, Tarragon, Verbena.

Disinfectant: Destroying germs.
Birch, Caraway, Clove, Dill, Juniper, Lime, Myrrh, Pine.

Diuretic: Increasing urine flow.
Angelica, Bay, Benzoin, Birch, Black Pepper, Carrot Seed, Cedarwood, Celery, Chamomile, Cypress, Eucalyptus, Fennel, Galbanum, Garlic, Geranium, Guaiacwood, Hyssop, Juniper, Lavender, Lemon, Lemongrass, Linden Blossom, Parsley, Patchouli, Pine, Rose, Rosemary, Sage, Sandalwood, Terebinth, Violet, Yarrow.

Emetic: Induces vomiting.
Violet, Rose.

Emmenagogue: Promotes and regularises menstrual flow.
Angelica, Basil, Bay, Caraway, Carrot Seed, Chamomile, Cinnamon, Clary Sage, Cumin, Fennel, Galbanum, Hyssop, Jasmine, Juniper, Lavender, Marjoram, Myrrh, Nutmeg, Origanum, Parsley, Peppermint, Rose, Rosemary, Sage, Santolina, Tarragon, Thyme.

Emollient: Soothing and softening skin.
Cedarwood, Chamomile, Geranium, Immortelle, Jasmine, Lavender, Linden Blossom, Mandarin, Rose, Sandalwood, Tagetes, Tangerine, Verbena.

Escharotic: Treating warts.
Cinnamon, Garlic, Lemon, Santolina.

Expectorant: Removing excess mucous from bronchial tubes.
Angelica, Basil, Benzoin, Bergamot, Cajuput, Cedarwood, Elemi, Fennel, Fir, Galbanum, Garlic, Ginger, Hyssop, Marjoram, Myrrh, Myrtle, Origanum, Parsley, Peppermint, Pint, Sandalwood, Ti-Tree, Thyme, Violet, Yarrow.

Febrifuge: Cooling and reducing high body temperature.
Basil, Bay, Bergamot, Cajuput, Camphor, Chamomile, Cypress, Eucalyptus, Garlic, Ginger, Hyssop, Lemon, Melissa, Niaouli, Orange, Palmarosa, Patchouli, Peppermint, Verbena.

Fungicide: Destroying fungal infections.
Cedarwood, Elemi, Garlic, Immortelle, Lavender, Lemongrass, Myrrh, Patchouli, Tagetes, Ti-Tree.

Galactagogue: Increasing secretion of milk.
Aniseed, Basil, Caraway, Cubeba, Dill, Fennel, Jasmine, Lemongrass, Litsea.

Haemostatic: Arrests bleeding/haemorrhage.
Cinnamon, Cypress, Geranium, Lemon, Lime, Rose, Terebinth.

Hepatic: Stimulates and aids function of liver and gall-bladder.
Angelica, Bay, Carrot Seed, Chamomile, Cypress, Grapefruit, Immortelle, Lemon, Origanum, Peppermint, Rose, Sage, Rosemary, Santolina, Verbena, Violet.

Hypertensive: Increasing blood pressure.
Camphor, Hyssop, Rosemary, Sage, Thyme.

Hypoglycemiant: Lowering blood sugar levels.
Eucalyptus, Garlic, Geranium.

Hypotensive: Lowering blood pressure.
Celery, Clary Sage, Garlic, Lavender, Lemon, Linden Blossom, Marjoram, Melissa, Tagetes, Ylang Ylang.

Insecticide: Killing insect pests.
Aniseed, Bay, Bergamot, Birch, Cajuput, Caraway, Cedarwood, Cinnamon, Citronella, Clove, Cypress, Eucalyptus, Fennel, Garlic, Geranium, Juniper, Lavender Spike, Lemon, Lemongrass, Lime, Litsea Cubeba, Myrtle, Niaouli, Origanum, Patchouli, Pine, Tagetes, Terebinth, Ti-Tree, Thyme.

Laxative: Aiding bowel evacuation.
Aniseed, Black Pepper, Camphor, Fennel, Ginger, Guaiacwood, Lemon, Marjoram, Nutmeg, Origanum, Parsley, Rose, Tarragon, Violet.

Nervine: Reduces nervous disorders.
Basil, Chamomile, Clary Sage, Hyssop, Juniper, Lavender, Linden Blossom, Marjoram, Melissa, Peppermint, Rosemary, Sandalwood, Vetivert.

Parasiticide: Ridding vegetable organisms living on other organisms.
Aniseed, Caraway, Cinnamon, Citronella, Clove, Cumin, Eucalyptus, Garlic, Lemon, Lemongrass, Myrtle, Origanum, Peppermint, Rosemary, Terebinth, Thyme.

Parturient: Helps easy delivery in childbirth.
Aniseed, Bay, Clary Sage, Clove, Dill, Jasmine, Juniper, Lavender, Nutmeg, Parsley, Rose, Spearmint.

Pectoral: Helpful for chest infections.
Cajuput, Fir, Hyssop, Violet.

Prophylactic: Helping to prevent disease.
Garlic, Hyssop, Lemongrass.

Resolvent: Dissolves boils and swellings.
Galbanum, Fennel, Garlic, Grapefruit, Rosemary.

Restorative: Restoring and reviving health.
Basil, Cypress, Lavender, Lime, Marjoram, Pine, Spearmint.

Rubifacient: Warming by increasing flow of blood.
Black Pepper, Camphor, Eucalyptus, Ginger, Juniper, Origanum, Pimento, Pine, Terebinth.

Sedative: Calming.
Benzoin, Bergamot, Cedarwood, Celery, Chamomile, Clary Sage, Cypress, Frankincense, Jasmine, Lavender, Linden Blossom, Mandarin, Marjoram, Melissa, Neroli, Petitgrain, Rose, Sage, Sandalwood, Verbena, Vetivert, Ylang Ylang.

Sialogogue: Inducing flow of saliva.
Cardamum, Cinnamon.

Splenetic: A tonic to the spleen.
Angelica, Chamomile, Clove, Fennel, Immortelle, Origanum, Lavender, Rose.

Stimulant: Increases flow of adrenaline and energy.
Angelica, Aniseed, Anise-Star, Basil, Bay, Black Pepper, Cajuput, Camphor, Caraway, Cardamum, Cinnamon, Citronella, Clove, Coriander, Cumin, Eucalyptus, Fennel, Ginger, Hyssop, Lemongrass, Niaouli, Nutmeg, Origanum, Peppermint, Pine, Rosemary, Spearmint, Tarragon, Thyme.

Stomachic: Relieves gastric disorders.
Angelica, Aniseed, Anise-Star, Basil, Bay, Bergamot, Black Pepper, Cardamum, Chamomile, Cinnamon, Clary Sage, Clove, Coriander, Dill, Fennel, Ginger, Hyssop, Juniper, Lemon, Melissa, Myrrh, Nutmeg, Orange, Origanum, Peppermint, Pimento, Rose, Rosemary, Santolina, Tangerine, Tarragon, Verbena.

Styptic: Arrests external bleeding.
Cypress, Lemon.

Sudorific: Increases perspiration.
Angelica, Basil, Cajuput, Camphor, Chamomile, Dill, Fennel, Garlic, Ginger, Melissa, Hyssop, Juniper, Lavender, Myrrh, Peppermint, Pine, Rosemary, Ti-Tree.

Tonic: Improves bodily performance.
Basil, Bergamot, Black Pepper, Cardamum, Carrot Seed, Clary Sage, Frankincense, Garlic, Geranium, Ginger, Grapefruit, Hyssop, Juniper, Lemon, Lemongrass, Lime, Mandarin, Marjoram, Melissa, Myrrh, Nutmeg, Neroli, Orange, Origanum, Parsley, Patchouli, Pimento, Pine, Rose, Rosemary, Rosewood, Sage, Sandalwood, Tangerine, Thyme, Verbena, Vetivert, Yarrow.

Uterine: Tonic to the uterus.
Clary Sage, Clove, Frankincense, Jasmine, Melissa, Myrrh, Rose.

Vascoconstrictor: Contraction of blood vessel walls.
Cypress, Geranium, Peppermint.

Vasodilator: Dilation of blood vessel walls.
Garlic.

Vermifuge: Expulsion of worms.
Basil, Bergamot, Cajuput, Camphor, Caraway, Carrot Seed, Chamomile, Cinnamon, Clove, Eucalyptus, Fennel, Garlic, Hyssop, Santolina, Lemon, Niaouli, Peppermint, Tarragon, Terebinth, Thyme.

Vulnerary: Prevents tissue degeneration and arrests bleeding in wounds.
Benzoin, Bergamot, Camphor, Chamomile, Elemi, Eucalyptus, Frankincense, Galbanum, Geranium, Hyssop, Juniper, Lavandin, Lavender, Marjoram, Myrrh, Niaouli, Origanum, Rosemary, Santolina, Tarragon.

Blends

Each of the oils in the groups below is said to blend well together, as well as to those in groups immediately adjacent.

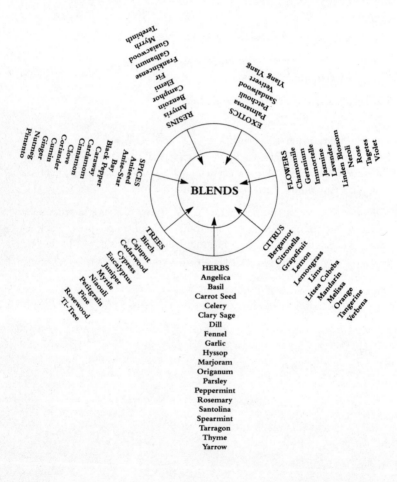

BLENDS

RESINS
Amyris
Benzoin
Camphor
Elemi
Fir
Frankincense
Galbanum
Guaiacwood
Myrrh
Terebinth

EXOTICS
Patchouli
Sandalwood
Vetivert
Ylang Ylang

SPICES
Aniseed
Anise-Star
Bay
Black Pepper
Caraway
Cardamon
Cinnamon
Clove
Coriander
Cumin
Ginger
Nutmeg
Pimento

FLOWERS
Chamomile
Geranium
Immortelle
Jasmine
Lavender
Linden Blossom
Neroli
Rose
Tagetes
Violet

TREES
Birch
Cajuput
Cedarwood
Cypress
Eucalyptus
Juniper
Myrtle
Niaouli
Petitgrain
Pine
Rosewood
Ti-Tree

CITRUS
Bergamot
Citronella
Grapefruit
Lemon
Lemongrass
Lime
Litsea Cubeba
Mandarin
Melissa
Orange
Tangerine
Verbena

HERBS
Angelica
Basil
Carrot Seed
Celery
Clary Sage
Dill
Fennel
Garlic
Hyssop
Marjoram
Origanum
Parsley
Peppermint
Rosemary
Santolina
Spearmint
Tarragon
Thyme
Yarrow

Essential Oils and
Skin Types

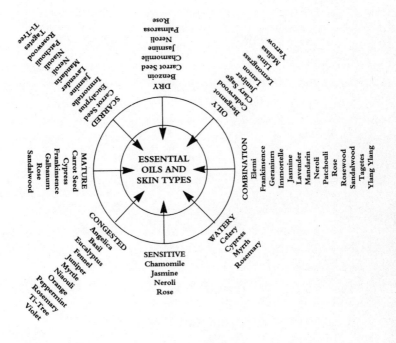

DRY
Benzoin
Carrot Seed
Chamomile
Jasmine
Neroli
Palmarosa
Rose

SCARRED
Carrot Seed
Eucalyptus
Immortelle
Lavender
Mandarin
Neroli
N'aouli
Patchouli
Rosewood
Tagetes
Ti-Tree

OILY
Bergamot
Cedarwood
Clary Sage
Juniper
Lemon
Lemongrass
Lime
Melissa
Yarrow

MATURE
Carrot Seed
Cypress
Frankinsence
Galbanum
Rose
Sandalwood

ESSENTIAL OILS AND SKIN TYPES

COMBINATION
Elemi
Frankinsence
Geranium
Immortelle
Jasmine
Lavender
Mandarin
Neroli
Patchouli
Rose
Rosewood
Sandalwood
Tagetes
Ylang Ylang

CONGESTED
Angelica
Basil
Eucalyptus
Fennel
Juniper
Myrtle
Niaouli
Orange
Peppermint
Rosemary
Ti-Tree
Violet

SENSITIVE
Chamomile
Jasmine
Neroli
Rose

WATERY
Celery
Cypress
Myrrh
Rosemary

SKIN TONIC
Angelica
Basil
Fennel
Frankinsence
Geranium

SCALP TONIC
Cedarwood
Chamomile
Clary Sage
Melissa
Rosemary
Ti-Tree
Yarrow
Ylang Ylang

Bibliography and Further Reading

The Essential Oils, Ernest Guenther Ph.D; D. Van Nostrand Co Ltd.

The Art of Aromatherapy; Robert Tisserand; The C.W. Daniel Co Ltd.

The Essential Oil Safety Manual, Robert Tisserand; The Association of Tisserand Aromatherapists.

Aromatherapy for Everyone, Robert Tisserand; Penguin.

The Aromatherapy Handbook, Daniele Ryman; The C.W. Daniel Co Ltd.

Lecture Notes on Essential Oils, David Williams MR Pharm S; Eve Taylor (London) Ltd.

Aromatherapy: The Use of Plant Essences in Healing, Raymond Lautie D.Sc & Andre Passebecq Md DPs; Thorsons Publishing Group.

The Best of Health: Thanks to Essentials Oils, Paul Duraffourd; La Vie Claire.

Aromatherapy, Judith Jackson; Dorling Kindersley.

Aromatherapy for Women, Maggie Tisserand; Thorsons Publishing Group.

Aromantics, Valerie Ann Worwood; Pan Books.

The Fragrant Pharmacy, Valerie Ann Worwood; Macmillan.

The Practice of Aromatherapy, Dr Jean Valnet; The C.W. Daniel Co Ltd.

Aromatherapy: An A–Z, Patricia Davis; The C.W. Daniel Co Ltd.

Subtle Aromatherapy, Patricia Davis; The C.W. Daniel Co Ltd.

The Power of Holistic Aromatherapy, Christine Stead; Javelin.

Practical Aromatherapy, Shirley Price; Thorsons Publishing Group.

Guide to Aromatherapy: The Secret of Life and Youth, Marguerite Maury; The C.W. Daniel Co Ltd.

Aromatherapy for the Whole Person, Dr Arnould Taylor; Stanley Thornes (Publishers) Ltd.

Herbs and Aromatherapy, Joannah Metcalfe; Webb & Bower.

Flower Essences and Vibrational Healing, Gurudas; Cassandra Press.

An Ancient Egyptian Herbal, Dr Lise Manniche; British Museum Publications.

The Herb Book, Elizabeth Peplow; W.H. Allen – London.

The Complete Book of Herbs and Spices, Claire Lowenfeld & Philippa Back; David & Charles (Pub) Ltd.

Beauty for Free, Catherine Palmer; Jonathan Cape.

The Complete Book of Herbs, Lesley Bremness; The National Trust.

Culpeper's Herbal, Edited: D. Potterton; W. Foulsham & Co Ltd.

Potter's New Cyclopaedia of Botanical Drugs and Preparations, R.C. Wren FLS; The C.W. Daniel Co Ltd.

The History of Herbal Plants, Richard Le Strange; Angus & Robertson Publishers.

The Concise Herbal Encyclopedia, Donald Law; John Bartholomew and Son Ltd.

Esoteric Psychology, Alice Bailey; Lucis Press.

The Greek Myths, Robert Graves; Pelican.

Periodicals: *Aromatherapy Quarterly, Aroma News, I.F.A. Newsletter* Common Scents (USA)